Praise for *The Stress Prescription*

"*The Stress Prescription* is an incredibly wise guide with simple, powerful advice. If you incorporate even one of these daily practices, it will lower your stress and boost your emotional well-being and health."
—Arianna Huffington, founder and CEO of Thrive Global

"The perfect prescription for this moment in time and outside of time."
—Jon Kabat-Zinn, founder of MBSR (mindfulness-based stress reduction) and author of *The Healing Power of Mindfulness* and *Mindfulness for All*

"A preeminent expert sheds light on how to handle the daily hassles of life. It's not just a manual for managing stress—it's a toolkit for preventing it."
—Adam Grant, #1 *New York Times* bestselling author of *Think Again*

"Elissa Epel reveals a welcomed truth: to master stress is not to avoid it but to move through it. With simplicity and wisdom, Epel teaches readers how to navigate stress with vibrancy, vitality, and joy."
—Esther Perel, psychotherapist, author, and host of *Where Should We Begin*

"Elissa Epel is *the* authority on stress and how we can transform it for good. She is a gifted teacher and translator of the mind-body mechanisms, making them accessible and useful."
—Daniel J. Siegel, MD, *New York Times* bestselling author of *IntraConnected*

"Elissa Epel, one of our foremost stress researchers, presents a richly researched yet practical and straightforward program for abating and preventing the many deleterious impacts of stress, a modern epidemic in our daily lives. In today's highly stressed and fractured society, this book is a salve for mind and body."

—Gabor Maté, MD, author of *The Myth of Normal*

"Most of us recognize that too much stress is harmful to our brains and bodies. The question is what can we do about it? *The Stress Prescription* has answers. Dr. Elissa Epel is both a brilliant researcher and a gifted communicator, breaking down the latest science into guidance we can trust. This book is a must-read!"

—Nadine Burke Harris, MD, MPH, former surgeon general of California and author of *The Deepest Well*

"This is really good medicine! Wise and practical, straightforward and truly helpful to all who want to reduce stress and live with more ease, *The Stress Prescription* shows us how to thrive amidst it all." —Jack Kornfield, PhD, author of *A Path with Heart*

"Dr. Elissa Epel's *The Stress Prescription* is for all of us. Reading it opens up the power to change the next moment from anxious to awe-inspiring, from fearful to fierce. Along the way, it delivers you to genuine possibility and potential whenever and wherever you need it most. Follow the good doctor's orders: These simple but profound research-driven practices just might radically change your life for good."

—Rhonda V. Magee, professor of law, University of San Francisco, and author and teacher of *The Inner Work of Racial Justice*

"Epel's decision to make this invaluable material available in such an accessible, practical, and impactful way for the public is a gift to us all. In *The Stress Prescription*, she reveals the often invisible forces that affect all of our lives, and guides us toward a healthier, happier, and longer life. This is a must-read for our new era of challenges."
—Richard Carmona, MD, MPH,
17th surgeon general of the United States

"*The Stress Prescription* is for everyone! Life is full of challenges and this book lays out in very practical terms how to navigate and flourish in the face of adversity. A compelling tapestry of personal stories, cutting-edge science, and the ancient wisdom of contemplative traditions, Elissa Epel does a brilliant job of weaving these elements together in a highly readable guide to flourishing in the modern world."
—Richard J. Davidson, PhD, *New York Times* bestselling author of *The Emotional Life of Your Brain*

"The compassionate and insightful writing in this book, combined with its highly accessible and practical guidance, make it a very valuable resource that will be used and appreciated by many in these uncertain times."
—Elizabeth Blackburn, PhD, Nobel laureate and *New York Times* bestselling coauthor of *The Telomere Effect*

"This book offers a powerful path out of stress and overload. Written by a renowned and compassionate scientist, the reader is offered both the science and methods for transforming stress as we face a world of uncertainty and increasing vulnerability."
—Roshi Joan Halifax, global humanitarian, founding abbot of Upaya Institute and Zen Center, and author of *Standing on the Edge*

"Elissa Epel is one of the most prominent stress scientists, with international stature. She connects research findings to what really matters to people in their everyday lives. In *The Stress Prescription*, Epel delivers practical, wise, sage, and transformative advice. The public needs this book desperately and Elissa is the only one could have written it."   —Robert H. Lustig, MD, MSL,
New York Times bestselling author of
The Hacking of the American Mind

"Whether it is personal crises, climate change and loss of biodiversity, or the many pains of inequality, we seem to be overpowered by the weight on our shoulders. Epel shows us that the only way forward is to discover and use the innate strength of our own shoulders, transforming the unbearable weight of stress into empowerment to live our best life."

—Christiana Figueres, author of *The Future We Choose*, former executive secretary of the UN Convention on Climate Change, and leader of the Paris Climate Agreement

"Stressful times call for de-stressing solutions. In *The Stress Prescription*, Dr. Elissa Epel, one of our nation's scientific experts on the biology and psychology of stress, provides practical guidance on reducing stress. Her prescription is also a recommendation for connection, a reminder that each of us holds the key to a less stressful world."   —Thomas Insel, MD, former director of the National Institute of Mental Health
and author of *Healing*

"This deceptively simple book actually holds sophisticated and novel keys to building stress resilience, all translated for you into concepts and tools you can use today. Get it for yourself, your staff, your patients, your kids—and change the impact of stress on your life for good." —Cassandra Vieten, PhD, executive director of the John W. Brick Mental Health Foundation, research scientist at University of California, San Diego

"Being human today is stressful. Period. While we can't escape the realities of the times we're in, we can find solace and practical advice through the wisdom in the pages of this book. Elissa Epel—scientist, teacher, and fellow traveler who cares deeply about humanity and the planet—is our trusted guide who shows us the difference one week can make in the rest of our lives."

—Susan Bauer-Wu, PhD, RN, president of the Mind & Life Institute, author of *Leaves Falling Gently*

"Managing today's adversities and traumas requires deep inner wisdom. In *The Stress Prescription* Dr. Elissa Epel has captured critical elements of this wisdom, leading us to understand the many ways we can listen to our body, learn and grow from our emotions, and connect with the inner peace and compassion that we each need. This book will be of great service!"

—Tsoknyi Rinpoche, renowned Nepalese Tibetan Buddhist teacher and author of *Open Heart, Open Mind*

"*The Stress Prescription* beautifully combines the rigor of science with the wisdom of reflection to offer a powerful and transformational roadmap for how to live a happier, healthier life. The wealth of ideas and practices presented in this illuminating work has the power to transform our individual and collective lives."

—Shauna Shapiro, PhD,
author of *Good Morning, I Love You*

"Simple, brilliant, and effective: world-class scientist Elissa Epel has done it again, helping us to feel better, live longer, and enjoy a resilient happiness. With personal stories, fascinating research, and many practical suggestions, you can feel her friendly support, cheering you on toward greater ease and well-being. This comprehensive guide is that rare book that is inviting and accessible as well as deep and far-reaching. It's grounded in its author's vast knowledge, deep personal practice, and heartfelt commitment to the welfare of others. This book is on my very short list of books someone should have if they're stuck on a desert island for the rest of their life. Truly a gem." —Rick Hanson, PhD, *New York Times* bestselling author of *Resilient*

PENGUIN LIFE

THE STRESS PRESCRIPTION

Dr. Elissa Epel is a professor and vice chair in the Department of Psychiatry and Behavioral Sciences at the University of California, San Francisco. She is an internationally renowned health psychologist who has conducted pioneering research into how stress impacts our health, all the way down to the cellular level. She is now focused on how to live well with existential stress, and ways to improve emotional well-being and to slow aging through personal and environmental changes. She was elected to the National Academy of Medicine, is the past president of the Academy of Behavioral Medicine Research, and is the director of mental health initiatives at the University of California Center for Climate, Health and Equity. She studied psychology and psychobiology at Stanford University (BA) and clinical and health psychology at Yale University (PhD). Her award-winning research has been featured in TEDMED, *The New York Times*, *The Wall Street Journal*, and many TV and science documentaries. Her first book, written with Nobel laureate Elizabeth Blackburn, *The Telomere Effect: A Revolutionary Approach to Living Younger, Healthier, Longer*, is a *New York Times* bestseller and has been translated into more than thirty languages. She loves the excitement of discovery research, the regenerative energy of collaborating on group projects, and the deep rest states and joy that come from nature and retreats.

THE STRESS PRESCRIPTION

Seven Days to More Joy and Ease

ELISSA EPEL, PhD

life

R_X

This book is dedicated to our ancestors, for the strength and resilience of their human spirit and the love through hard times that enabled us to be here, and to you, the reader, for your own often heroic efforts to live and love well through these uncertain times.

PENGUIN BOOKS
An imprint of Penguin Random House LLC
penguinrandomhouse.com

Copyright © 2022 by Elissa Epel
Penguin Random House supports copyright. Copyright fuels creativity, encourages diverse voices, promotes free speech, and creates a vibrant culture. Thank you for buying an authorized edition of this book and for complying with copyright laws by not reproducing, scanning, or distributing any part of it in any form without permission. You are supporting writers and allowing Penguin Random House to continue to publish books for every reader.

A Penguin Life Book

LIBRARY OF CONGRESS CATALOGING-IN-PUBLICATION DATA
Names: Epel, Elissa, author.
Title: The stress prescription : seven days to more joy and ease / Elissa Epel, PhD.
Description: New York : Penguin Books, [2022] | Includes bibliographical references.
Identifiers: LCCN 2022026840 (print) | LCCN 2022026841 (ebook) |
    ISBN 9780143136644 (trade paperback) | ISBN 9780525508144 (ebook)
Subjects: LCSH: Stress (Psychology) | Stress management. | Mental health.
Classification: LCC BF575.S75 E64 2022 (print) | LCC BF575.S75 (ebook) |
    DDC 155.9/042—dc23/eng/20220613
LC record available at https://lccn.loc.gov/2022026840
LC ebook record available at https://lccn.loc.gov/2022026841

Printed in the United States of America
1st Printing

Book design by Daniel Lagin

Some names and identifying characteristics have been changed to protect the privacy of the individuals involved.

Neither the publisher nor the author is engaged in rendering professional advice or services to the individual reader. The ideas, procedures, and suggestions contained in this book are not intended as a substitute for consulting with your physician. All matters regarding your health require medical supervision. Neither the author nor the publisher shall be liable or responsible for any loss or damage allegedly arising from any information or suggestion in this book.

CONTENTS

INTRODUCTION

EXPECT THE UNEXPECTED

WOULD YOU LIKE TO LIVE IN A WORLD WITH NO STRESS?

Picture it: No worry. No anxiety. No pressure.

Sound nice?

Maybe for a moment. But *stress* is woven into our experience of life so deeply, so essentially, that entangling it from life itself is impossible. As tough as stress can be to cope with sometimes, we would be a lot worse off without it. Humans have a stress response for a reason: it prepares our mind and body for what we need to do in the moment and in the moments ahead. Evolutionarily, our body's natural stress response saved our prehistoric lives time and again. It's the reason we're here today, and we still rely on it to motivate us. To give us a surge of energy and clarity. To deliver the physical and mental resources we need to meet a challenge. And a healthy, "peak-and-recovery" stress response—where we experience a shot of stress and then recover quickly afterward—is actually good for the body. We humans are exquisitely built to handle stress. In fact, we *need* it.

In the right dosage and frequency, it helps keep our cells young and vital.

But these days, most of us do have a stress problem.

We're "turned on" to stress all the time. Stress is the ocean we swim in. From the moment our eyes open in the morning to when they drift closed at night, we are flooded with constant stress triggers: demands and deadlines, logistics, to-do lists, unexpected crises both small and large, thorny conversations. There are so many triggers that can set off your body's stress response, activating that potent cocktail of stress hormones that courses through your bloodstream and affects everything from how fast your heart beats to how you digest your food and store fat to how you think. Even our own thoughts become stressors that our bodies respond to. In fact, our thoughts are actually the most common form of stress.

So what do we do?

We can't eliminate stress. It will always be a part of life—anything worth doing will have aspects of stress woven throughout: challenge, discomfort, risk. We can't change that. But what we *can* change is our response to stress. And in a rapidly changing, unpredictable world, we can do this with a beautifully simple pivot: we can learn to expect the unexpected.

When the Unexpected Happens

Bryan Koffman, my neighbor, is in his fifties. He and his wife, Yana, live down the street from me in a quiet, leafy neighborhood in San Francisco. He works with elderly residents in a long-term care facility. He enjoys his work, the city where he lives, his marriage. If you asked him, he would say, "Life is good." But his life wasn't always so stable and fulfilling.

Bryan grew up in Russia. He married young; at age twenty, he was a newlywed just starting out in his career. He wanted to become a nurse. Instead, he was drafted into the Soviet Army and sent to an arctic base.

He was devastated. He had to leave behind his school, his career, and his family for a two-year training stint in an area of the country that was fifty degrees below zero, where he could die if he didn't secure his protective gear properly. He was losing everything that mattered to him—he might even lose his life. Not everyone survived the training, and after, there was a high chance he would be deployed to Afghanistan.

The stakes were high. It felt like there was nothing to gain and everything to lose. His anxiety levels, he says, were off the charts. Not knowing what would happen, feeling completely out of control—his nervous system was fired up all the time.

Chronic Stress Is Toxic Stress in the Body

Even if you've never been deployed to the arctic tundra, my guess is Bryan's stress feels familiar. Stress isn't inherently bad. But chronic stress is. I study stress and its impact on well-being and aging. I've looked at stress under the microscope, investigating how it can change the structure of our very cells, right down to our telomeres, the "caps" at the ends of our chromosomes that turn out to be important biological markers of health and aging—microscopic "clocks" hidden inside each of our cells. And what I've seen is this: Chronic stress, the type that goes on for years and years, has a toxic effect on your body. It wears out your cells prematurely.

A lot of the advice we get about how to deal with the stress in our lives is good, but incomplete: Get rid of stressors. Learn strategies to relax. To those I say, absolutely! These are great first steps. And in fact, in this book I offer effective strategies for both reducing stressful situations and truly relaxing. But there's a big caveat. First, you can't eliminate all stressors—not even close. Stress is interwoven into even the most joyful and fulfilling aspects of our lives: everything from parenting to career growth to reaching for big life dreams can be very stressful. These things are stressful because we care a lot about them. We can't just stop caring—nor do we want to. And second, many strategies for relaxation end up being quick fixes, Band-Aids, that don't really help you in the long term. When the next wave of stress comes along, it's just as overwhelming as ever.

I told you stress can be a good thing. But *chronic* stress doesn't do anything good for you. It's only damaging. There's a whole litany of health ramifications of chronic stress that we could go through—like increased risk of obesity, heart disease, diabetes, depression, and dementia—but the main thing to understand is that chronic stress gets into your cells. Chronic stress leads to elevated blood levels of the triad of important stress factors—cortisol, oxidative stress, and inflammation. And when these are ever present inside your cells, your telomeres—those protective caps at the ends of your chromosomes—get worn down. They get shorter faster. Why does this matter? Because critically short telomeres damage our mitochondria, the batteries in our cells that give us energy and keep our cells healthy. And worse, when a worn-out cell reaches the end of its healthy life, it enters a harmful and irreversible state of old age (called *replicative senescence*).[1] Fortunately, we can turn things around before they reach that state.

Many of the tissues in your body must regenerate to stay healthy, meaning you must create new cells. This regeneration has to happen in critical areas in the body like immune cells, the cells of your cardiovascular lining, and the hippocampus, the area in the brain that is so vital for memory and mood. And it turns out that telomere length is ultimately what determines how long a cell can keep dividing. The longer your telomeres, the more times your cells can divide, replicate themselves, and refresh tissues. When they get too short, this can no longer happen. The cell becomes senescent—it stops replenishing. The cell dies or spews out inflammation. It's at the end of its road.

Having short telomeres in our blood cells predicts earlier onset of diseases and death. So we take this issue seriously. People often ask me if telomere length is more a *marker* of aging (like a cellular "record" that reflects age) or a *mechanism* of aging (a causal part of the aging process). The answer is both. If you have a genetic propensity for long telomeres, it directly predicts lower rates of chronic illnesses of aging like heart disease, showing telomeres have a mechanistic role. Chronic stress can lead to early aging through many pathways, and telomeres are one of the mechanisms. When chronic stress leads to worn-down telomeres and inflammation, it *causes* premature aging, through that process of creating dysfunctional senescent cells that I've described.

This is a big concern for me as a stress researcher. Because when we're too stressed for too long, it accelerates biological aging, and disease develops early. And the research shows that on average, our stress levels are only increasing.

Super Stressed

The COVID-19 pandemic caused a dramatic spike in depression and anxiety, but our stress levels as a population had already been on the rise for years. Stress researchers have been tracking people's days, asking them about stressful events that occurred and how they felt afterward. They have found that over the past twenty years, people have experienced more frequent stressful events, and further, they have felt more stressed out by them.[2]

The intensity of our stress is going up.

Usually we think that stress happens only when there is a stressful event—like, say, getting drafted into the Soviet Army! That's an extreme one, and big events like breakups or loss definitely drive up stress levels over months. But daily occurrences—like encountering traffic in your commute—also spike your stress response. Stress researchers often focus on stressful events, but it may be far more telling to focus on how relaxed or vigilant one is under normal circumstances, at baseline, to see how we are holding on to stress in our minds. So let's talk about the state we spend most of our time in: our default stress baseline.

The stress response is pretty straightforward. When we sense a threat cue from the environment, our bodies process the cue and send alarm signals to the brain. But what about when there is no salient, obvious threat looming, when there is uncertainty in the air—what does the brain do then?

We are wired to survive, to look for danger, to be vigilant, because the world—whether ancient jungles or modern cities— has always been full of uncertainty and danger. When we are in this default mode, our brain searches for cues of safety and certainty, and the process depletes the glucose energy in our brains.[3] It is like always being set on high battery mode. Uncertainty has a cascade effect in our brain, cuing first the anterior cortex and then the amygdala (the fear center), which then activates our stress response networks. In this high battery mode, stress spreads through our whole body at a low level, all the time—just in case something happens. But when things are certain, and we feel safe and can relax, we can switch to "low battery mode" and conserve energy. Unfortunately, most of the time, our hardworking, certainty-seeking brains are running on high.

Where's Your Baseline?

Most of us try to cope with stress by relaxing or by avoiding distressing thoughts and feelings. These are not robust solutions to our pernicious modern stresses. They are simply not enough. Even if we can "relax" back to baseline, our typical level of baseline is too high. We need to be able to reset our baseline *lower* so that when we come down from our stress response, we can truly recover and restore.

We are not typically "at rest." And when we are resting, it's not very deep. There is a state that is better than our usual relaxation, and more rare: deep rest. When we can get there, it's biologically restorative. But with a stress baseline that's too high, this state is virtually out of reach.

MIND STATES CREATE PHYSIOLOGICAL STRESS OR RESTORATION

STRESS AROUSAL

RESTORATION

RED MIND (acute stress)

YELLOW MIND (baseline cognitive load)

GREEN MIND (rest)

BLUE MIND (deep rest)

MIND STATES

The human nervous system has an incredible range. Unfortunately, it's often "stuck" at too high a level. Our research team at the University of California, San Francisco (UCSF), with Alexandra Crosswell, PhD, leading, has mapped out the spectrum of "mind states" available to us, and we have identified the "deep rest" state that so many of us are missing as critical to stress resilience and well-being.[4] Let's take a look, starting at the top left of the preceding graph:

Acute stress (red mind): A stressful event happens, and we are triggered to "red alert." The body mounts the acute stress response; for some, thoughts go to catastrophic. This acute stress response *can* be healthy—if it's short-lived. Red mind means we prioritize creating energy over everything else—we release glucose galore; we are ready to run.

Cognitive load (yellow mind): On a typical day, our level of arousal is here. It's lower than acute stress, so we think it is our baseline resting state, but this is nowhere close to rest. Our "cognitive load," the amount of information the brain is trying to hold on to all at once in our limited memory bank, is typically still quite high. Here's the thing about yellow mind: When we are done with work, or when nothing stressful is in front of us, we may still be experiencing stress arousal in the body. We may still be creating stressors with threatening or strongly negative thoughts. And even more pervasive: we might not even be aware of stressful thoughts. Researchers have pinned this high state of arousal to unconsciously feeling unsafe. This is especially true when we feel lonely, low status, or discriminated against, or have had childhood traumas that make us expect an unsafe environment.[5] But any of us can be propelled into this state of chronic multisensory overload from subtle and unconscious uncertainty stress. Plus, we're often dealing with multiple sources of stimulation, including negative information and demands coming in from screens, and we don't help ourselves with the multitasking we typically do. For most of us, our default baseline—how stressed we generally feel—is in this yellow mind state, in the stress arousal zone far above relaxation.

Rest (green mind): This is a pleasant state of relaxation that can occur while we're passively engaged in leisure activities or when our attention is fully absorbed in actively performing tasks we enjoy, sometimes called the "flow" state. It also describes when we are just *being*, and not being asked to do something. Rather, we are in a receptive state, such as observing nature, beauty, art, or entertainment. The common theme here is that we are monotasking, not multitasking, and feeling ease and safety. These kinds of activities, among others, are known to activate the vagus nerve, which travels from the base of the brain stem all the way down the body. Vagus nerve activation helps trigger a state of relaxation in the body, and over time increases *vagal tone*, which helps us recover from stress more quickly. The more time we can spend in a state of rest or deep rest, the more we are training our nervous system to live in a more restorative mode.

Deep rest (blue mind): This is a deep state of restoration that is cultivated by changing our environment from one of stimulation to one of quiet and safety. Typically, this means physical seclusion, and either narrowing our attentional focus or having an open drifting focus of attention. Blue mind states, when the body is at its lowest level of psychological and physiological stress arousal, develop during deeply relaxing activities such as mind-body practices or meditation, and do not typically last long. Blue mind is when true body restoration, like cell regeneration, can take place. The stage of deep sleep, the most restorative stage for our bodies, is also a time of deep rest.

To sum up, we are living most of our life in the red and yellow mind states. We rarely access green, much less blue mind states. Our mission, as part of the Stress Prescription, is to push our default baseline level closer to true rest. To live well with stress, we need to drop our default baseline.

Becoming Stress Resilient

We know now that stress biology and aging biology are wrapped up together. Our bodies get worn down more quickly under chronic stress, and chronic uncertainty is the most ubiquitous chronic stress. Thus, the antidote: We need to "turn off" our threat response to uncertainty. We need to shift our mindset to *accept* uncertainty as the defining condition of our lives, instead of fighting against it or feeling threatened by it.

At that arctic army base in Russia, my friend Bryan had a turning point. He realized that most of what was causing him anxiety and stress about his situation was completely out of his control. He didn't have a choice to be there or not; he had to stay. He couldn't control when he woke up, or when he ate, or what he did with his time. In the midst of this tremendous overhaul of his life, buffeted by uncontrollable forces, he had a shift in perspective. *I can view this differently.* Fighting his current reality in his head was taking away any chance he had at feeling joy. While his peers were feeling extreme anxiety, he realized there was a gift in having no choice. The weight that had been crushing him suddenly lifted.

He started to focus on the simple comforts that existed in his day. Small things became meaningful; he felt he was connecting with others more deeply. When he had a day of leave in a nearby town, he felt pure elation at the freedom to choose his meals, to talk to new people, even simply to pay his bus fare. Earlier, he'd given up writing letters home, because whatever he wrote was openly read and often censored. But he decided to start writing home again anyway, about positive things that wouldn't be censored. There were more positive things to find— even in his extreme situation—than he'd realized, once he started looking for them. Now, he actually recalls this as a period when he most experienced bliss in his life, the joy of being alive and appreciating it.

Luckily, Bryan was not sent to Afghanistan. When his two years of training were over, he was able to return home. But he never forgot the experience and the way that mental shift helped him through.

During the first year of the COVID-19 pandemic, Bryan's wife, Yana, suffered from anxiety and worry about everything: their eldercare business (Would the residents get COVID?), people she loved (Would their son drop out of college?). Her busy mind was expert at scanning for potential catastrophes. Bryan, on the other hand, was comfortable with the uncertainty and lack of control.

"Why are you buying cans of beans and reams of toilet paper?" he would ask her, with an incredulous but loving smile.

Bryan knows—on a deep level—that life is defined by uncertainty. That many things are beyond our control. But he also knows that he can get through a challenge. He knows how to find joy and be at rest, even in a stressful, uncertain world. If he could live well, enjoy his life, and find moments of rest and calm as a young soldier in the bitter arctic, he could do it anywhere. There are events that stress him out, of course—he's not a robot! But it's not uncertainty of the future that gets to him.

Those who practice Buddhism know a core tenet is accepting impermanence—that everything changes and nothing lasts, including our own lives—which helps them embrace this challenge of uncertainty. When I had the chance to interview His

Holiness the Dalai Lama about how to deal with crises, I asked how we can be more comfortable with uncertainty. His answer was immediate.

"As far as uncertainty is concerned, in Buddhist beliefs, things are always changing and the future is unpredictable. Some of the problems we face arise naturally, but now a lot of the problems we face, like climate change, are problems of our own creation." He then discussed the need to expect uncertainty, and train our hearts and minds for remaining calm, clearheaded, and warmhearted.[6]

That's why this week, our overarching goal is to *expect the unexpected*. We are going to learn to combat stress by being flexible, open, and present-focused.

Expecting the unexpected is a mental shift that makes us feel okay when things go awry, or simply not as we've envisioned. It allows us to more comfortably bear the ambiguity and uncertainty of life. If we expect the unexpected, when the unexpected does happen, we *don't* have an overexaggerated and prolonged fight-or-flight response. Our heart does not thump. Our body doesn't tense in response to the "threat." The data show that the more we can accept and exist comfortably with uncertainty, the less likely we are to develop chronic stress, anxiety, depression, or PTSD when times get hard. The more resilient we'll be to ongoing, unpredictable stressors like, say, pandemics or natural disasters. The faster we recover from traumatic stressors. And the more we can go out and live our lives more fully.

We all have different starting points, from genetics to our

personal histories to our current life circumstances, that establish our "stress profile." We've been shaped by our genetics and our pasts. But we also have neuroplasticity, the brain's remarkable ability to form or reorganize neural connections if we repeat new thoughts or behaviors over and over. We can tweak our experiences and shape our brain responses toward more flexibility and tranquility. We can train our minds and bodies for greater stress resilience so that we can live longer, healthier lives that we can enjoy for the time that we're here.

HOW TO USE THIS BOOK

WITHIN THE PAGES THAT FOLLOW ARE THE LIGHT AND PORTABLE ESsentials you need for an era of uncertainty. There is so much we can't control. But we *can*, to a great extent, control our reactions to the curveballs life throws at us. With some relatively simple new habits, we can train the mind and body to experience the inevitable stresses of life in a positive way that is actually healthy for the body.

Over the course of this book, we are going to learn to:

- Embrace uncertainty.
- Put down the weight of what we can't control.
- Use our stress response to help overcome challenges.
- Train our cells to "metabolize stress" better.
- Immerse ourselves in nature to recalibrate our nervous system.
- Practice deep restoration.
- Fill our busy schedules with moments of joy.

All of this will give us the resources and resilience we need to face the uncertainty of life—to ride the waves instead of getting pulled underneath them.

When the wildfires swept through California in the fall of 2020, they got close to where I live. I remember packing a go bag of essentials—it needed to be light and portable, everything in it useful and essential, stuff you can easily carry and use immediately. That was a literal go bag, but what we need now is a metaphorical go bag with real tools to handle the uncertainty and stress we face in life. So that's what this book is going to be.

This book offers a seven-day plan to transform your relationship to stress. Each day is designed to give you one new skill—a tool to put in your metaphorical backpack—that will stay with you as you move forward. These practices need no special equipment, and at most take five to ten minutes. Can you make a difference in your stress levels in a single day?

Yes.

A single day can be very influential. It's a unit of time we have a lot of control over. We frame our life around the day. It's where we do the work of worrying and of self-care. It's where we establish the patterns and routines that determine our well-being. With small adjustments, you can make an enormous difference in how you experience your life.

Approach this book, and each practice, with 100 percent self-kindness, flexibility, and forgiveness. If you don't have the bandwidth to read this book in a week, then don't. What we don't want to do is *create more stress*. You can read a chapter a day or a chapter a week. You can take breaks and repeat practices for however many days you wish before moving on. You can move through this book at whatever pace is right for you. Your job is to figure out how to fit this into your busy life so it adds joy, not stress. If you ultimately adopt even one daily practice regularly, you will have made a big difference in your well-being. That is success.

What I hope you will end up with after our time together: a nimble, flexible mindset, new knowledge and insights about your own stress responses and nervous system, and the tools to manage them well for joy and healthy longevity.

THINGS WILL GO WRONG . . . AND THAT'S ALL RIGHT

THE STUDY WAS NOT GOING WELL.

It was a year into the COVID-19 pandemic. Conditions for everyone, everywhere, were unpredictable: Would there be another lockdown? Would the new variants spread? Would schools reopen as planned? Inside our lab, things were just as shaky. Participants and lab staff got sick and disappeared into quarantine. Supply chain disruptions meant we suddenly lacked critical pieces of equipment that had filled the drawers and cupboards pre-COVID.

"We're out of pipette tips?" I remember saying in utter disbelief to one of our lab assistants. Without this simple piece of plastic, we couldn't perform some of the most basic procedures. Labs all over the country were pipette-less due to supply chain issues.

The studies we were running felt particularly urgent: we were examining pandemic depression and COVID-19 vaccinations through a grant from the National Institutes of Health (NIH). The vaccines were proving to be highly effective—hopeful news and surely reason for optimism. But what about in the longer term? How long would antibodies last? What factors might help or hinder the body's process of maintaining antibodies against this virus? With other vaccines, we know that personal habits like poor sleep, smoking, and high psychological stress can dampen our response to vaccinations. Clearly, many of us felt pummeled by pandemic stressors, and that might mean fewer antibodies. With the herd immunity of an entire planet in question, we wanted to know: Could psychological well-being, like feeling daily joy and purpose, protect us from stress and lead to a stronger immune response?

In a study like this one, we have to find out more about people's lives and how they think, how much joy and angst they experience on a typical day. Participants complete daily surveys designed to show us what they found stressful and the degree to which they felt stressed. What was the most stressful thing that happened to you today? How long did you think about it after? Was it a minor hassle, like traffic, or a big thing, like a major conflict with a partner? Combined with the physiological data, the answers to these questions paint an invaluable portrait of each person's stress profile. And it helps us understand how expectations shape stress. One of the questions we ask everyone is: How predictable is your day?

Everyone wants predictability. As humans, we are wired to want it. We long to anticipate what will happen to us moment to moment, to plan around stable landmarks in our day and in our year. Our bodies want lunch to happen when lunch is supposed to happen. When we pull out of our driveways, our brains want our routes to work or school to be the same as they were yesterday (and no traffic!). When our environments are mostly predictable, we feel safer. We can relax, to a certain degree, even with other stressful events on our plates.

We each have our unique starting baseline—the level of stress arousal that we usually hover around through any typical day. Every person's starting baseline is different: some people are tightly wound up, vigilant, and ready to startle at an unexpected noise, while others might be like a placid lake that is hard to disturb. Regardless of where we start from, the lower we can get our baseline stress arousal, the better—it means we'll be much more able to tolerate the peaks of stressful events. But when our baseline is already high and things don't go as planned—when the unexpected comes flying at us—that already high baseline spikes even higher. *Fast.*

I'd put a lot of my personal and professional life on hold for our COVID study. It required all of my time and bandwidth. I had an away message up on my email that shocked people (*Sorry, I am not available*), and had stopped taking requests for talks. My study codirector, Aric, and I were working on this project around the clock, coordinating lab assistants, ensuring that all the administrative safety precautions and paperwork were done, workshopping study protocols, and responding to every crisis that popped up. I was so invested in the study running smoothly and proceeding according to schedule for the NIH that everything that went wrong felt like an attack. And things *kept* going wrong.

When we schedule one participant, to draw their blood and measure their stress response, we need a full, coordinated team

., a lab tech, and a whole pack of researchers. So
)ne canceled, it was a big deal. And almost every
. One week, some of our staff could not come in
fires that were raging on the West Coast had
driven them from their homes. A few days later, the smoke from
the California fires turned the San Francisco skies an apocalyptic
brick red. The air quality monitors bounced over to dark purple,
the worst possible rating on the scale. On top of that came . . . a
heat wave. But we could not open our windows to escape the heat,
because the smoke was so bad. On several days, we had to shut
down the lab and pause the study completely.

I found myself tense with worry about what would be the
next emergency, the next wildfire, the next thing to go wrong.
Meanwhile, I'm a stress researcher. I've been studying stress
and its impacts on health and aging for almost thirty years. I
knew that uncertainty stress, which was exactly what I was experiencing, is one of the most pernicious forms of chronic stress
out there. Because it is subtle, quiet, and pervasive, it's something we often don't notice that we've habituated to, over
months or years. In particularly uncertain times, it's easy to
jack up our default baseline state toward higher stress arousal.
This type of stress can stay with us while we rest and even while
we sleep, if we don't attend to it.

The Price of Vigilance

The human brain loves certainty. It's what allows our nervous
system to relax. When conditions are predictable and stable, we

have more cognitive bandwidth to spend on thinking, problem-solving, creativity. Our mental real estate isn't being sucked up by planning, wondering, worrying, and catastrophizing about what *might* happen. But uncertainty, in recent years, has become one of the defining circumstances of our lives, and it takes a biological toll on our bodies.

When what's going to happen next is a question mark, we respond to it physiologically the way our ancestors might have responded to a vast, open plain: exposed and vulnerable, we go on high alert. Physically, the body shifts into a prepared state, readiness for fight or flight. Subtle shifts happen—heart rate goes up slightly, muscles tense (but not necessarily in a perceptible way). Undercover, our body is working harder in this pre-stress state waiting for the big *something* to happen. The mind and body have entered a vigilant state of readiness—not only scanning for danger, but *expecting* it. We are engulfed in the invisible stress of uncertainty.

Obviously, in a prehistoric survival situation, this kind of mental stance would be hugely advantageous. This tendency of our stress response to fire up in reaction to an uncertain or ambiguous situation certainly saved our *Homo sapiens* hides a million times over and is part of the reason we're still here as a species. And our stress response to rapidly developing situations can still be a huge boon for us in terms of being able to fire on all cylinders when we need to: The cortisol that your hypothalamus releases into the bloodstream makes glucose more available in the body. Glucose is a type of sugar—it translates to energy. We actually know what chronic anticipation stress can do to a cell: In a groundbreaking new study, my colleague Martin Picard of Columbia University tested the effect of chronic exposure to cortisol on the life span of cells. The cells were in a sense on red alert, anticipating threats, all the time. Their metabolism increased: in other words, they went into high battery mode. As a result, they had dramatic telomere shortening, replicated fewer times, and died earlier.[1]

When you're going into a short-term situation that comes with uncertainty—for example, giving a speech or presentation—you can really use that burst of mental and physical energy. But what's so interesting, and problematic, about uncertainty is that it's pervasive. It isn't limited to a few distinct moments in your day or week. It's everywhere. It's *What bad thing will happen next in this study I'm running?* But it's bigger than that— *What will happen in my life? What will happen for my child? What will happen for the country, the economy, the planet?*

And further, it's hidden from us. Overt stressors are often quite obvious, like red flags waving. We can see them, prepare for them, and then recover after (more on this later). Uncertainty is subtle. Without our conscious choice, we—all of us—are devoting a certain amount of subconscious attention to scanning for danger, not only through our waking hours but during our sleeping time as well. We are in a neurobiological state of vigilant attention—and we don't even realize it. This is yellow mind.

The healthy ideal for our bodies is a balance between activity of the sympathetic nervous system (fight or flight) and the parasympathetic nervous system (rest and digest). But uncertainty stress leaves us with perpetually elevated sympathetic nervous system activation. We never get the chance to recover. With a mindset that is intolerant of uncertainty, we are in a state of chronic stress.

Uncertainty Tolerance Is a Skill We Need to Build

Uncertainty affects not only our mood and stress, but even our decision-making process. One study asked participants to play a simple computer game in which certain outcomes (like finding a snake under a rock) might cause a mild electric shock on the hand. But the researchers varied the outcomes: some participants never received the shock, some received it half the time, and the final group always got the shock. It turned out that the people who experienced the most uncertainty—the ones who got the buzz *half* the time—experienced the most psychological stress. Their sympathetic nervous system (fight or flight) was on high vigilance, heart rate increased, pupils dilated. It wasn't the shock itself that spiked stress—it was the *uncertainty*. And, interestingly, those in the uncertain condition performed the worst in the game and took longer to make decisions.[2]

In our study on stress and vaccination responses, we measured people's level of uncertainty tolerance to see how much it impacted stress responses during the pandemic. Just as we thought: those with lower tolerance tended to have much higher levels of post-traumatic stress from the pandemic, experiencing more intrusive thoughts, avoidance, and anxiety over time. Another pandemic study found those with less tolerance of uncertainty did more panic buying of goods such as toilet paper and canned food.[3] Meanwhile, we know that the more we are able to tolerate uncertainty, the less we are prone to more serious psychological conditions—higher uncertainty tolerance is associated with lower rates of anxiety and depression. Those with anxiety are particularly affected by uncertainty: they tend to have a cognitive bias of seeing danger when there's ambiguity, and will often respond to an uncertain situation with a full-on threat response.[4]

Like most things, uncertainty tolerance runs on a spectrum—some may cope reasonably well in the "open space" of ambiguity, with nervous systems that are simply better calibrated to those types of conditions; others really struggle and are much more reactive. A whirlwind of various factors could be determining your uncertainty tolerance, including genetics, upbringing, personality, and life experiences. One study with mice showed how a specific set of neurons in the limbic system creates anxious behavior when there is an environment that feels uncertain.[5] Mice instinctively gravitate toward small, dark spaces for protection and perceive wide-open spaces as inherently threatening—understandable, because in the wild the chance of their getting scooped up by a predator is fairly high. In the study, when the mice were out in the open, specific neurons in the memory and emotion area of their brain were activated—neurons that overpowered "higher order" problem-solving and thinking—and triggered knee-jerk avoidance behavior in the mice, who scurried back to the shadows. But when the research team figured out how to essentially turn off those "anxiety neurons," the mice relaxed and began to explore the open space.

The point is not that healthy rational caution is never called for—if we turned off all the anxiety neurons in every mouse out there, they would become dinner for owls. The point is that we can draw a direct line from uncertainty to anxiety to a full threat response, and finally to avoidance of anything uncertain or ambiguous. People who tend to be high on intolerance of uncertainty experience much more anxiety and stress. In the extreme, the clinical profile shows that when people cannot tolerate even a tiny amount of risk (and they often view ambiguity as risky), it becomes what we label "generalized anxiety disorder," which is characterized by having your attention stuck in "scanning for danger" mode, worrying excessively, and presenting with physical anxiety symptoms (excessive worry, avoidance of new situations, tense body, startle responses). People with generalized anxiety disorder tend to seek reassurance over and over, and to avoid ambiguous, "open field" situations. But when we're avoidant of situations that contain a bit of uncertainty, we cut ourselves off from a lot of life experiences and opportunities. We are the mice; life is the owl.

My friend Cheryl is a vigilant scanner. I'm pretty confident she's high on intolerance of uncertainty. When our children were young and we would stroll with them through the neighborhood, she would often suddenly gasp and cry out, "Where's Debbie?" Debbie was never far.

I knew why she had such a strong startle response and high vigilance: she had been through her share of traumatic experiences in the past, and her nervous system was wired tightly. Now, even twenty years after the difficult events she went through, she still has a powerful "alarm system" inside her that constantly goes off when it doesn't need to.

Our kids are grown, but we still walk our dogs together. She has an app on her phone called Citizen—whenever there's an incident anywhere in the city, at any time, she gets a notification. Her phone buzzes, she pulls it out, and she reads, "Three miles away, on Sherwood Court, there was a break-in." We laugh about her app, but once I asked her why she uses it.

"I know it's a silly habit, and it does make me worry," she replied, "but it gives me a sense of control."

A sense of control can help us with stress—and we are going to talk about that in the next chapter. But constant vigilance will keep us in the far-from-restful yellow mind state of stress arousal. The better strategy is to work on getting comfortable with uncertainty—acclimating your nervous system to the reality of not knowing everything, and being okay with that. When we are good at tolerating uncertainty, we are more likely to trust others, cooperate, and collaborate.[6] And whether we are liberal or conservative, we are less likely to hold rigid, highly polarized political views (a major source of stress!).[7]

Finally, Cheryl has deleted the crime-alerting app and feels it was a good move—it helps her do a little less constant scanning. Some of us may always have a stronger automatic stress response, and we might not be able to radically change that. What we can do is change what we do *next*. So wherever you fall on the uncertainty tolerance spectrum, know this: *You can move the needle.* You can become more tolerant of uncertainty in your day, in your life, and in your future.

The "Violation of Expectation" Effect and How to Beat It

Vivian and her adult daughter, Alicia, talk on the phone every day. Though they live across the country from each other—Vivian in San Francisco and Alicia in New York—they are quite close. Vivian loves that she and her daughter have managed to remain in touch so regularly, despite being so far apart geographically, and she has a real sense of the texture of Alicia's days. But she does notice something. Their chats always seem to end with Alicia venting about how upset she is over something that didn't go as expected that day. To Vivian, it's striking that Alicia seems equally distressed by all of the events she describes—trouble finding parking on an outing, for instance, seems to upset her just as much as a teacher expressing concern that her child may have ADHD. Alicia often dwells on how well things had been going that day before the incident. She has a favorite phrase she always deploys at the end of these tales of plans gone awry: "It's always something!"

Vivian is baffled by this. "Well, of course it is," she always says. "Why would you expect anything different?"

Vivian finds herself wondering: How did they end up with such different mindsets? In her mind, this is just how life is; there's no reason to believe anything will go smoothly. As she was growing up, her family moved around a lot, and she learned quickly to adapt and make the best of each new situation. When her own daughter was born, Vivian wanted to make things more stable for her. She even passed up an opportunity or two because it would have meant uprooting her family, and she wanted Alicia to have more consistency than she'd had. But now she wondered—had she given Alicia the impression that the world could be controlled, predicted, made to fit your plans and expectations? In washing away some of the difficulties she faced, had she failed to set her daughter up for the way life *actually* unfolded? Vivian expected detours and construction; Alicia expected straight routes, green lights, and smooth sailing.

Vivian is a friend—not a study participant. I've never pulled her into the lab to draw her blood, review her stress surveys, or peer into her cells. But if I did, and if I compared them with her daughter's, I wonder what I would see. It's possible that as Vivian and Alicia move along through the years, their calendar age staying stable at thirty-two years apart, their biological age is actually closing the gap. Vivian, who rolls flexibly with the kicks and punches her days throw at her, doesn't seem to mount a stress response when faced with an unexpected detour. Alicia has a completely different physiological response to that ROAD CLOSED sign. Her sympathetic nervous system whooshes into action, ready to fight this threat. And if that's happening a lot— all day, every day—that's not good.

When things go awry, we tend to react with a stress response. In Buddhism, this is thought of as the second arrow problem: Anytime something bad happens, it's like we're being hit by two arrows. The first arrow is the painful thing that happened; the second is our reaction to that bad thing. In other words, problems (the first arrow) are inevitable, but suffering (the second arrow) is optional. The events will happen. The first arrows fall on everyone. But if we *suffer about the suffering*, we are throwing a second arrow at ourselves, and it's always a double hitter. For Alicia, this was in part because of a "violation of expectations." Alicia thought, *Why me?* Vivian had a different response: *Why* not *me?*

We are always visualizing and imagining how the rest of our day, week, or even life will go or should go. The human brain has an incredible capacity to visualize possible outcomes. We do it effortlessly, often without even consciously realizing we're doing it. We visualize lunch: outside, on the park bench in the sun. We visualize the afternoon meeting, and what we'll say if we're put on the spot. We visualize the future: getting the job we applied for. And then when these expectations are violated, it's easy to feel like a tragedy has occurred. Like we have been wronged. Like we are a victim. But there is a way to keep dreaming about the future, without living in chronic red mind states.

Loosen Up Expectations

Going into our COVID study, I had some pretty firm expectations of how it would all turn out based on how our previous studies had gone: The cupboards would be stocked with the supplies we needed. We would have enough staff. Participants would appear as planned. I didn't think about the fact that I had these expectations—but they were there, and every time they were subverted, I *did* feel threatened. With every unexpected incident, I felt that surge of adrenaline, the racing heart, the mind scrambling around to figure out, *What now?*

It was my colleague Aric, who led the study with me, who reframed it for me. After an exhausting week full of glitches and crises, the last straw for me: a participant lost her biosensor ring . . . because her house had burned down. Suddenly I was doubting all our research efforts. I thought, *This participant just experienced one of the most traumatic events possible, and so will others. We never should have launched this study! We should all be at the wildfire evacuation shelters helping out.* I thought about throwing up my hands and giving the grant money back. But Aric just calmly pointed out that the trend of the study had been for things to go wrong, not right. Why would we expect it to suddenly be different?

It was true! With pandemic supply disruptions, staff and volunteers canceling due to COVID exposure or loss of child-care, wildfires continuing to cut off roads, and forced evacuations, we could only expect more of the same. For the remainder of the study, I woke up each morning with an attitude of openness to whatever was going to happen that day—even another crisis. When something went wrong, we just shrugged. "On brand," we would say. We'd reached a new point where we *expected* something to go wrong, so that when it did, we could roll with the punches. And when things surprised us and went smoothly, we felt appreciative and grateful. In short: I had accepted the absolute uncertainty of each day, so it was no longer a threat to me.

So today, as you begin shifting your own stress resp[e] number-one thing I want you to do is to realize that thi[s] go wrong this week, and that's okay. By "wrong," I don't neces-sarily mean "bad." I mean not according to your expectations. Strong expectations can hurt us whether they're positive (something we're looking forward to) or negative (something we're dreading). Better to loosen our expectations as much as we can.

A Present-Centered Mindset Is a Nimble, Flexible Mindset

My yoga teacher says, "Expectations rule out the possibility of being present." Because you're projecting into the future, you are no longer here, right now. And *here* is the only place you can actually experience certainty.

I'm not going to tell you to never have expectations of what may happen in your day or your life. Our brains are prediction machines—we do it automatically, all the time. It's not realistic to try to renounce expectations altogether; we need to imagine and dream. But our expectations become a problem when we get too attached to them. The solution is not to stop having ex-pectations, but to *notice* when we have strong expectations, smile at them, and to remind ourselves not to get attached—to be ready to let them dissolve.

As stress researchers, when we evaluate classes that may help people manage stress better, we test how much people improve in their well-being, and also how long those improvements last. And one thing we know now is that some techniques (certain types of breathing, high-intensity interval exercise) are effective, but the benefits fade if you don't continue the specific practice. Meanwhile, meditation or mindfulness interventions that are based on cultivating a present-centered mindset have longer-lasting effects . . . even when you're *not* practicing them every day.

My colleagues and I ran a study in which we recruited women who had never meditated before, and split them into two groups. The control group was sent on a one-week vacation at a luxury resort where they could swim, take walks, and relax. The other group stayed at the same resort—but for eight hours a day they practiced mantra meditation, yoga, and self-reflection exercises. We wanted to know: Does a long, relaxing break mitigate stress just as much as contemplative practices? Or does meditation really do something more?

At the end of the week, everybody had indeed benefited—all the women felt fabulous. They reported dramatic improvements in feelings of vitality as well as decreases in stress and depression. (No surprise, really, that the human nervous system does well at a beautiful resort, whether you're meditating or not!) But when we followed up almost one year later, the groups had diverged in their well-being. The control group had bounced right back up to their pre-vacation levels of stress and depression—it was as though the break had never happened. Meanwhile, the meditation group had actually maintained their lower levels of stress and depression a year later. Some of the women had kept

up the practice, but that didn't fully explain the positiv
across the group. We think that even a short meditatic
ing can leave us with a different mental filter, a new awareness
of how our mind works, and the capacity to recognize our
thoughts as just thoughts—fleeting observations rather than
real events or true statements—draining them of their power to
trigger an unnecessary stress response. This ability to observe
our mind is called *metacognition*.

Meditation has long been part of my own stress-management
plan. I don't always find the time for a daily meditation practice, but at least once a year, I try to make it to a retreat where
I can practice being present and embodied, and I experience
the residual effects of these retreats for quite a while afterward. I do find, however, that the transition from the deep rest
state I can reach retreat and back to my daily fast-paced, high-
stress life can be sharp and jarring. Leaving one retreat I at-
tended, I got into the driver's seat of my car, buckled up, turned
the key in the ignition, and suddenly felt my mind whir into
action right along with the car engine. I'd been calm and cen-
tered moments before. Then I was fully immersed in anticipatory planning mode on high speed: projecting into the rest
of the day, thinking about the next task, and the one after
that; I had five things on my to-do list already, and the familiar race against time was on. My body was tensing up: *What's
next?*

I turned the car off and called the meditation teacher I'd just
spent the weekend with.

"I just lost everything we've been practicing all week!" I

said. "It feels like a switch flipped in my brain as soon as I left. I'm back to those type A tendencies."

"Okay," she said. "Pause for a moment. Check your body. Are you leaning forward?"

I was.

"That's what we're doing with the mind," she continued, "when we get caught up in the whirlwind of planning. So right now, I want you to physically lean back. And *mentally* lean back. Let experience come to you. Let time unfold moment by moment, let it meet you wherever your body is at. Our bodies can't time travel. Use your body to ground you here now."

I leaned back and breathed more slowly. I was delighted to find that it helped.

We spend so much time forward projecting—trying to plan, trying to iron out uncertainty. Sure, we need to figure out the logistics of our days. But it's very easy to tip over the line from productive planning into wheel spinning that wears us out, tanks our mood, and creates vigilance in our body. What I learned that day is that body posture is a great antidote to this. Leaning forward, we are telling our mind to choose the future over the present; we can become radically disembodied and no longer feel where we are. Leaning back, we bring our mind back to our body; now grounded in the present, we can experience the certainty of *this* moment.

"But what about being prepared for potential problems?" you might ask. "Isn't it better to have a plan for how you'd respond?" Well, even if something negative does happen as you predict, you can easily worsen your response to it by anticipating it all day. One study found that when people were anticipating upcoming stressors, it spiked negative emotions, just like a real; no surprises there. But later, if the event did actually occur, they were no more resilient to it than they would have been without all those mental aerobics—they had just as big a stress response as they did to events they did not anticipate.[8] In other words, the worry didn't help them one bit. One of our own studies found that people under chronic stress anticipated and reacted to an upcoming task before they even started it, and the earlier their cortisol spiked, the greater their levels of oxidative stress over the next hour.[9]

Anticipating problems isn't helpful. It ramps up our stress response and increases the likelihood that we'll have a negative experience during the challenging event we were trying to prepare for. So instead of holding on to expectations about how things will unfold, try practicing "I don't know" mind—an open state of curiosity, humility, and neutrality. When you embrace "I don't know," you stop clinging to an outcome, you drop the narrative of catastrophic outcomes, and you open yourself up to the range of possible outcomes. When you answer someone with "I don't know" (genuine, not snarky!), you will likely get a surprised smile back. For me, during that 2020 study, the "not knowing" mind worked as a kind of armor. I feel now that I have a more prepared mindset for the next pandemic—or whatever it will be.

Today you're going to ask yourself: *Do I feel uncertain about things right now? Do I have rigid expectations about the future?* And then you're going to loosen those expectations. You're going to remind yourself: today is a wide-open field of possibilities.

Today and before each practice, you will see this image of a wave below. This is your visual reminder to lean back, take a long, slow breath, and welcome a new experience.

TODAY'S PRACTICE

CATCH AND RELEASE

Go-Bag Skill: Embracing Uncertainty and Openness

Today we practice relaxing into moments of uncertainty, instead of tensing up against them. Uncertainty often shows up as *embodied stress*, which is when we turn stress and negative emotions into feelings, sensations, and tension in the body. Thankfully, our physical sensations can also shape our emotions; by letting go of tensions in our bodies, we can change our emotional state.

To begin, find a place to sit, if you aren't sitting already. Ideally this is someplace quiet and comfortable, but you can do this anywhere, even on the subway or bus, or at your desk at work. (If you can, put earbuds in to block out distractions or listen to calming music.) Next, follow the steps below.

- **Tune in to your body.** Close your eyes. Ground yourself: take three slow breaths, all the way down into your belly. Briefly, notice the physical sensations you're experiencing right now: the feeling of the chair you're sitting on, the temperature of the room.
- **Scan for embodied stress.** For about sixty seconds, slowly scan your body with the flashlight of your attention, starting at the top of your head and gradually moving

down to your toes. Stress lives in the body, but we all carry it in different places. Notice where you're holding tension—neck, shoulders, lower back? Release it. If your hands are clenched, open them. If your shoulders are tensed, roll them back. Breathe into any remaining tight or heavy spots—that's where you're holding uncertainty.

- **Now, ask yourself:**
  - What's on your mind right now, as you think about the day ahead, the week ahead, or the future in general?
  - What are you feeling most uncertain about?
  - What expectations are you holding about how things will go?

- **Let go of expectations.** Notice strong attachments to how you think things should go, and see them for what they are: one *possible outcome*, not a sure thing. Mentally wipe clean the whiteboard of the day or week ahead. Remind yourself that anything can happen, including unexpected positive things. Uncertainty is welcome. Now you've named it, smile at it; breathe into it. That's the unknown, the unpredictable, the mystery that will unfold with time.

- **And finally, lean back.** Lean back physically in your chair. When you are more reclined in your seat, you're more receptive, relaxed, and open to what's coming. Recline comfortably and match your mental stance to the ease of your body's posture. Let experience unfold and come to you, moment by moment, savoring the certainty of *this* moment. In this moment, you are safe. You can relax.

Bonus Practice

Uncertainty stress tends to creep up on us. For extra credit, catch uncertainty stress as it settles into your body during your day.

- **Choose three times today to catch embodied uncertainty stress:** Set a timer on your phone to go off at those times. Make it a pretty chime or bell.
- **When the timer goes off:** Pause whatever you're doing and smile: time to check in with your body! Find a place to sit, and repeat the preceding exercise—What are you uncertain about right now? Scan the body to find any stress and tension, and release it.
- **Anytime today you find yourself tensing up:** That may be unconscious stress you can make conscious, by naming it, and then you can release it. Close your eyes, lean back, and focus on your breathing. Welcome a warm feeling of open receptivity to this moment. Remember that uncertainty about the future (even five minutes from now!) is a given. Anytime you want, you can tap into the present moment and experience the certainty and ease of this moment, *right now*.

Troubleshooting

Sometimes we're worried about something and just can't stop. Giving up the feeling of control is difficult, so first and foremost, don't be hard on yourself. Some of us, particularly those of us with early childhood trauma, have developed pretty strong habits of mind that don't allow us to feel safe easily, to experience the meaning of "let go." If you find you cannot just stop whirring and churning on something, here are a few options to try.

1. Make a realistic assessment of the probability of risk.

If you're worried about something that might happen, game it out. What's the worst that could happen? And what's the likelihood that this actually comes to pass? With everything in life, there's some risk, but often it's extremely low. Focus on what's *probable*, not what's *possible*.

For people with serious anxiety, often called generalized anxiety disorder, chronic worry can be debilitating. But strategies from cognitive behavioral therapy can help reduce worry and free people to engage more in life. Try setting up small uncertainty experiments: Take a problem (for example, wanting to be social but feeling anxious about going to a party), and make a prediction (*When I go to the party, I will not have anyone to talk to; I will sit alone*). Could you live through that experience? Most likely, yes. Do the experiment and write down what happens. You have flexed your uncertainty muscle. Repeat and build the muscle. You will get more accurate data on how often the most feared outcome happens. (Much less than you think!)

2. Make a plan . . . and then set it aside.

The urge to plan is sometimes a sign that you do need to do a little mental prep so you can feel prepared and relaxed later. So go ahead and do it. But then stop—don't keep planning in your head! Once you are in the stressful situation, you need to be able to *be* in that moment, to see the situation as it really is (not as you imagined it to be), in order to be effective. A present-centered mindset is a nimble, resilient mindset: plan for a situation concretely, but then put the list down. Then you can be here now.

Personally, as someone recovering from a strong need for control, I have developed a lifelong habit of making a to-do list and putting it aside, as part of my nightly wind-down ritual. That way I don't spend sleep time reciting my list or adding to it, trying to control the future.

3. If it's world news that's intruding . . .

You aren't an island or in a bubble. The world has become a highly uncertain place to live, and its events affect us. These days, we all consume a lot of news. During the last election, I wanted to know what was happening every minute. I was constantly checking news sites. I felt exhausted yet slept terribly. Sometimes I'd check the news in the middle of the night!

Too much media—particularly during disasters—is actually a major highway to post-traumatic stress symptoms.[10]

This is a well-researched phenomenon: when we watch news stories during crises, we feel worse, not better. A study done after 9/11 found that the people who viewed the most media, especially visual images, developed more anxiety symptoms and health issues up to three years later.[11] Now, in an increasingly interconnected world, most of us can access the news at all times. But the science-based truth is that we shouldn't! Constant checking is *not* a good way to deal with uncertainty about the world.

Ask yourself: *Does checking now help, or can it wait?* The news never stops. There's always something you could be checking on. In reality we rarely need news in real time. When you feel the urge to check on something, tell yourself, *Later. The news will be there later.*

CONTROL WHAT YOU CAN . . . AND PUT DOWN THE REST

JANE HAD JUST TURNED FORTY-FIVE. AN EVENT PLANNER, SHE HAD been derailed by a bout of depression, something she'd struggled with since she was a teenager. Generally, she knew how to manage it: therapy and medication. This time, she didn't catch it fast enough. She was already in the swirl of it before she realized she needed help. And by then, she'd lost her job at an upscale restaurant, along with her steady income. The city she lived in was expensive—she'd been living month to month and had no savings.

She moved in with her mother, who lived an hour outside the city and had a spare room. It would just be temporary until she got back on track. She found a new event planner job, but it was only part-time corporate catering and felt like a step down. Meanwhile, bills mounted, and she felt constant stress over not being able to save. How would she ever move out?

And then, the unthinkable happened: her mother had a stroke.

At the hospital, the MRI results were not encouraging. With physical therapy, the doctors said, Jane's mother could recover some of her functionality, but many of her limitations would be permanent. Jane's capable, relatively young mom was, in the blink of an eye, incapacitated.

Fast-forward a couple of months: Jane's mother has recovered quite a lot—in fact, more than the doctors thought she would. With the help of a walker, she can move around. Her speech is pretty good. Her snappy sense of humor is back, and she's doing most of the things she enjoyed before the stroke. But she has right-side weakness in her leg and hand. She can't cook for herself, and Jane worries about her falling while she's at work. But her mother doesn't want to have outside help come in, and Jane no longer feels she can move out—at least not unless her mother improves, but the doctors haven't given them any clarity on how likely that is, if at all. Meanwhile, at work, Jane is getting panicky about things that never fazed her before. Missing silverware right before an event. A billing error. Sometimes she feels like she spends the whole day with her heart in her throat. Everything just feels completely out of control.

A sense of control is one of the pivotal factors that drives our stress levels up and down. We *love* control. As we learned in the previous chapter, the human brain desires predictability. We want to know our future. And not only to *know* it, but to have the power to determine how it unfolds to the greatest extent possible. Feeling "in control" can reduce stress, especially chronic toxic stress: you still encounter stressful events, of course, but when you have a sense of power over your day, you are more equipped to experience a healthy peak-and-recovery stress response, with a quick return to baseline, that *benefits* your mind and body. Meanwhile, a person who feels they have no say in the flow of their day, their work, or important conditions of their life may experience the opposite in response to the same type of stressors: a threat response that peaks but never resolves; a constant, chronic state of stress born of uncertainty and powerlessness.

A high sense of perceived control in life is associated with being happy, healthy, and wealthy.[1] Feeling in control of our lives helps us regulate emotions and be more resilient. For example, when we feel more control, we have lower emotional reactivity to stressful things that may happen at work, at home, or in our social networks.[2] After a stressful event, people with a high sense of perceived control not only feel less anxious but also have fewer physical symptoms, like headaches, stomachaches, or pain. And the more perceived control people feel over their lives, the more frequently and intensely they feel positive emotions, and the less frequently and intensely they feel negative emotions. A sense of control enhances our emotional stability. And, some good news for the AARP crowd: older people in particular are protected from the negative effects of high stress by a feeling of control—this was true even during COVID.[3]

But control is a mixed bag. Yes, a sense of control can give us a feeling of power instead of powerlessness, driving down fear, anxiety, and stress. But when we try to control the uncontrollable, the opposite happens.

Control: A Double-Edged Sword

When it comes to managing stress, we need to be able to feel a real sense of control when we can, but also *know* what's beyond our influence to change. A natural response to the uncertainty of life is to attempt to exert more control in order to make your world more predictable and therefore "safer." When things feel like they're slipping from our fingers, the instinct is to grip tighter. But trying to exert our will over situations that are beyond our influence only makes stress constant and therefore toxic.

An interesting study on baboons illustrates this perfectly, and holds lessons for humans as well—we're a lot like baboons in clothes. We are both highly social creatures, and social stratifications affect our health. Baboons are hierarchical primates, where dominant males control everything from interactions between subordinates to general resources. Due to their status and capacity to control their environment, male and female baboons who are dominant benefit: their health is better overall, and they tend to have less cardiovascular disease.[4]

When the hierarchy becomes unstable for males, however, things change. Baboon social hierarchies can get disrupted by death, extreme weather or other environmental changes, conflicts with other groups, and conflict within the group. When former alpha males are no longer living in the same stable, predictable environment as before—for example, when they're moved to a new enclosure and they find themselves in new social groups, needing to assert themselves—their physiological advantage evaporates along with their position of power. They develop more cardiovascular disease than subordinates. But the problem is not just that they no longer have the control they once did. It's that they continue to try to control things. They are hardwired to do it, but it's like they're throwing themselves against a brick wall. And they pay the price: higher stress hormones and more illness.[5]

Control is great when you have it, but if you're striving for it and can't achieve it, you suffer. Control is a double-edged sword: it can work as a tactic when you have a stable, predictable environment, but not when you don't. And as we discussed in the previous chapter, "predictable" can be swept away at any moment. We have a predictable environment—until suddenly, for any number of reasons, we don't.

One of the biggest unpredictable disruptions we can experience in our modern lives is illness. If you've ever had to care for a loved one with a serious illness, you have probably felt helpless about their condition. I've studied caregivers extensively over the course of my career. I'm particularly interested in understanding the experience of caregivers in my stress studies because there are a lot of factors they can't control about their lives. For our stress health studies, we enroll family caregivers (versus paid caregivers), because this type of uncontrollable and unrelenting stress adds up over years and can start to affect health. My colleague Janice Kiecolt-Glaser and her late husband, Ron Glaser, conducted classic studies here, showing, for example, that caregivers have wounds that repair and heal more slowly, taking nine extra days for complete healing.[6]

After studying caregiving for many years, and being a caregiver myself, I know that the issue of control matters a lot. Caregivers of family members with mental illness have a particularly tough path: They experience conditions that alarm the amygdala, the part of the brain related to emotions, like feeling overwhelmed, burdened, and trapped. Their finances are affected by costs of care and by lost productivity and income. They have higher rates of depression, anxiety, and healthcare usage.[7] So on top of that, to survive, they need to focus on the little they *can* control, to maximize their stress resilience.

The question "What can I control?" is an urgent one for caregivers. You want to advocate for your loved one. You want to get them the support and interventions they need in order to thrive. At the same time, you can't change medical conditions or genetic disorders. And you can't predict their trajectory. With any diagnosis, a lot about the future (both theirs and yours) becomes uncertain. The challenge for caregivers in this situation is to learn how to support without trying to control—figuring out where to pour their love and energy into research or action that will help without spinning their wheels or trying to move a mountain that will never be moved.

It's a process of constant mental calibration, and it's not unique to caregiving or parenthood. The same applies to caring about someone with addiction, also not something you can control, or when we become deeply invested in service and making change, as with careers in activism, medicine, and social services. In any situation where we care deeply about the outcome, it's easy to get swept up in a long battle against the uncontrollable. But so often, it's a fight you cannot win: you will not be able to achieve the control you seek; meanwhile, your own health will suffer.

What we have to learn to do in these types of life situations is separate the circumstances of our lives into two buckets: what we *can* control and what we *can't*. For a long time, I kept a quote from the Dalai Lama pinned to my refrigerator door:

> If a problem is fixable, if a situation is such that you can do something about it, then there is no need to worry.
>
> If it's not fixable, then there is no help in worrying.

Today, we're going to work on this: control what you can, and put down the rest.

Something that can help you immediately is to become more aware of where your mental energy is going. You have limited bandwidth; attention is a precious limited resource. Notice when you're spending a lot of time anticipating something that hasn't happened, or ruminating about something that already has. When something is sucking up your mental bandwidth, ask yourself: *Is this something that's in my control?*

Remember my friend Bryan, whom we met at the beginning of this book? His moment of epiphany—when he realized he was struggling against the uncontrollable—was pivotal for him. He'd accepted what he could not control, focused on the little

ould, and consequently experienced an immense sense
lom. This epiphany transformed into a form of resil-
improving his well-being and his capacity for joy. With
his attention focused on the small daily things he *could* control,
he felt that the sensory world had opened up to him, and he
could experience the richness of life in a new way. He felt fully
alive and could appreciate that. He connected with people more
deeply and felt he could read their emotions more vividly. This
sense of bliss lasted for several months, and he never forgot
what it felt like. It seems paradoxical that this was one of the
most stress-free times of his life. But there is a lesson here. If we
focused on the things we can control, and accepted everything
else, what would our days be like?

Let's Take Inventory

Often, what we're chafing against is something we have very
little control over, if any: A child's behavior or diagnosis. Another
person's opinion or treatment of you. A problem that someone
we love is struggling with. The outcome of elections. And even
what nature has in store for us: fires, floods, extreme weather,
pandemics. We spend a lot of energy on situations we cannot
change. In an attempt to control the uncontrollable, our bodies
mount a "take-action" stress response that gets us nowhere yet
keeps the stress baseline elevated.

So today, we're going to sort your major stressors into two
buckets:

1. What I have the power to change
2. What I cannot change

In the previous chapter, we talked about the vagueness of uncertainty stress: the way it becomes so pervasive, we no longer realize that it's sapping our resources—both physical and cognitive. We worked on catch and release: catching ourselves in those moments of stress and letting it go. Now, we build on this. We're going to take a good, clear look at the stressors in your life.

Stressors look different for each of us. We all perceive the world through a unique lens that's shaped by our past experiences, genetics, and more. One person might find commuting to work stressful, while another person might love the alone time. **Take a moment and follow the instructions for the Stress Inventory in the box below.**

STRESS INVENTORY

Grab a pen and paper (or better yet, a notebook for keeping track) and write down everything you can think of, right now, that causes you to feel pressure, stress, anger, or uncertainty. You might think about your daily routine, relationships, and work. Be as comprehensive and detailed as you can. One important note: don't try to think about solutions right now. Your job is simply to get every stressor you can think of down on paper.

that you've taken inventory, look at that list. The first
we're going to do is see if there's anything you can delete,
like pruning branches. Something all of us should be doing,
from time to time, is to look at our Stress Inventory and ask: *Do
I need to keep this?* One way we can exert control is to set down
something and say no.

Delete Stress

We feel out of control when we have too many balls in the air.
Sometimes, the right thing to do is to let some of those balls
drop.

The most common reaction I hear in response to that advice
from people is that they *can't* drop any of the balls. Everything
is necessary. Everything is critical. People depend on them.
Nothing can give. But it's essential that we interrogate these
beliefs.

Several times a year, I offer mindfulness retreats for the general public—one of my favorite things to do is to translate the
mind-body science into resources that people can use and I lead
this exercise at the retreats. After hearing the predictable answer that they are stuck with the list of situations, I ask them to
question, deeply, whether that's actually true. The reality is,
you simply can't do it all. You need to find something to give up.
Take stock of what you're carrying: Is there anything you can
put down, at least for a while? Is there anything you can completely let go of?

It's not always easy to see what we can get rid of or take a break from. If it's on your plate, you put it there for a reason. It's job related. Family related. It doesn't seem optional. But sometimes what we need to do is zoom out and take a really broad perspective, to ask ourselves these hard questions:

CAN I PUSH THE DELETE BUTTON?

In the long run, how much does this specific activity matter?

Who says this is required, and is that really true? Whose voice do I hear?

What would actually happen if I got out of this situation or responsibility? Or delegated it?

Is there a way to taper it off slowly?

What's the worst thing that might happen? Could I live with that?

And what benefit would there be?

For a lot of people, work commitments are the hardest. People feel obliged to say yes to responsibilities out of a desire for approval or advancement, pressure, wanting to be a team player, or fear of losing their jobs. But if you're stretched thin, it's especially important to consider ways to politely decline requests and set stricter boundaries. Sometimes, setting boundaries at work can be seen as a sign of strength—colleagues may respect your time more and pile less on you to begin with. Learning to say no at work is an incredibly valuable skill. Of course, every work environment is different. There are places where saying no—however graciously—is simply, and unfortunately, not part of the culture. If you're in a work environment where saying no is not tolerated, it might be worth exploring whether there are healthier conditions in other companies or industries.

An ideal workplace improves our well-being. In reality, the conditions for burnout are baked into many work cultures—and then work detracts from our health. It's the demands of the job matched with poor resources or understaffing, not some personal failure that causes work burnout. Burnout is a pernicious form of chronic stress—it's the constant demands over years, without time for recovery. This leads to a toxic and cyclical triad—emotional exhaustion, feelings of cynicism, and feeling you are ineffective and can't perform well. You can barely get through each day. Your internal rhythms for sleep and hormones can get dysregulated—cortisol can become either too high or in some cases too low.[8] So the only true solutions are changing your coping *and* your work conditions, and when it's not possible to improve the work conditions, leaving the job.

Women often do more of the hidden work, including service-oriented work, that does not get recognized, and then experience higher burnout. Dr. Christina Maslach, the pioneer on burnout research, has identified critical ingredients that protect from burnout: supportive colleagues, some control over decisions and workload, feeling appreciated and recognized for your work, feeling things are fair and equitable, and finding meaning in your work.[9] I've realized that reducing daily time pressure, simply slowing down, is critical for living well—allowing more moments for embodied presence, gratitude, restoration, and seeing people as their whole instead of as part of a work transaction. Constant time urgency is a culprit in reducing the quality of our days—and carving out even just a couple of minutes between tasks to take a few conscious breaths, welcome your next meeting, and set positive intentions can help.

Social commitments are also tough. We want to show up for the important people in our lives. But often, we get overwhelmed with a deluge of social obligations that become more of a drain than a source of fulfillment. Yes, community is very important. People with strong social networks have smaller stress responses. But a strong social network doesn't necessarily mean a big social network. We see through studies and surveys that as we age, we prune our social circle to be smaller because as our time on this planet grows a bit shorter, we find that we are no longer willing to invest in relationships that aren't supportive and satisfying, that have significant negatives. The question we can all ask ourselves is: *Why wait to prune back my social network so that it's more positive and supportive? Why not prioritize positive relationships now?*

By no means is this a directive to let go of friends who are going through a hard time. Sometimes relationships become tilted in one direction or the other; sometimes you lean on someone, and later they lean on you. No relationship will ever be perfectly balanced forever. When you zoom out on your life to look at where you can cut back on pressures and responsibilities, take the long view. It will also help you refocus on who is most important in your life, and where you want to put your time and energy. This kind of perspective taking may make it easier to "delete" stressors that are cluttering your day now.

Think about it this way: taking away some of those things will help you *add back* time that you otherwise wouldn't get with someone you love.

A lot of us, especially those who use social media, have this FOMO—fear of missing out. We say yes because we don't want to miss anything. We want to go to all the things. We want to be part of the group, to keep up. But all these things you're feeling pressure to join aren't necessarily things that are going to keep your social ties thriving—not if you're feeling stretched thin and brittle. Sometimes the best thing you can do for your well-being, your relationships, and your capacity to handle the stress in your life is to say no.

Simplify Your Day

The COVID-19 pandemic was an interesting lesson in this exact thing. When the lockdowns struck in March 2020, we were all forced to withdraw from the world in possibly the most sudden and extreme way any of us had ever experienced. For many, jobs were suddenly remote. Their social networks spiraled closed to include only members of their households, or even just themselves. Some people weathered months of the pandemic completely alone. One friend I Zoomed with that year said, "I haven't touched another human being in six months." By the time vaccines were available and the extreme social distancing could soften, most of us were champing at the bit to reengage with the world, to "go back to normal." But at the same time, an interesting phenomenon was happening. Many suddenly felt reluctant to simply pick up where they had left off. People paused. Some of the things they'd thought of as "required" pre-pandemic were now, quite clearly, not so obligatory after all. Reengagement became an opportunity to evaluate the various facets of our lives and to ask: *Do I really need this? Does it need me? I have limited attention and time—is this where I want to place it?*

Maybe we didn't want to put all this stuff right back on our plate. Maybe we wanted to reengage with the world in a way that was more aligned with our passions and values. Suddenly, here was this chance to ask ourselves: *What kind of life do I want to be living? And does all this stuff align with that?*

We don't need a global pandemic to sweep through our lives in order to do this kind of "taking stock" a bit more frequently. Often we aren't prompted to take a healthy, wide-angle perspective on our lives until something big happens. Sometimes it's a major birthday in midlife. Other times it's something much sadder, like losing someone. Whatever causes it, it shocks us out of the narrow, nose-to-the-grindstone perspective we tend to take out of necessity—to get everything done, to stay on track. But that "track" we're on can slowly, over time, veer off course. And if we don't pick up our heads every so often and look around, we can find ourselves a long way away from where we thought we were going. Every time we say yes to something, we are leaving less time for the things we may care about more. When you look at your weekly schedule, can you refine your time use?

This is big-picture stuff I'm talking about, and today, of course, is just one day. You're not going to reevaluate your entire life today—don't worry! When we study stress, we look at the big brushstrokes of people's lives, the general conditions that add stress, like low control at work or excessive caretaking responsibilities; and the factors that reduce stress, like an optimistic view or feeling a strong sense of purpose in life. But we also look at daily habits, the building blocks of our health; the effects of our daily routines are additive and magnified over time. Within our habits, our routines, our day-to-day schedules, is the aggregate of our lives. It's easy to say, *I'll take something off my plate next month*, but try not to put it off too long: as the writer Annie Dillard eloquently puts it, "How we spend our days is of course how we spend our lives. What we do with this hour or that one is what we are doing."[10]

To determine whether you can delete stress by taking something (or several things) off your plate, you may need to look at your day today, and your week ahead, and really ask yourself: *Is everything I'm doing aligned with what's most important to me?* In answering this question, you can get valuable clarity on what must stay (even if stressful) and what can go.

What Really Matters?

A powerful way to figure out what you can delete, and where to focus your energy, is to *work backward from death*.

A friend and colleague of mine, Martica Hall, who was living under a terminal cancer diagnosis, recently gathered up all of the people who'd been important to her over her life and career—friends, research partners, former students—for a group phone call to say goodbye. She was in hospice at that point, and was told that she was very likely at the end of her life. It was shocking news; we all struggled to come to grips with the suddenness of it. I was nervous to get on the call, but once the group call started, my anxiety drained away. It ended up being an incredible hour of joy and laughter as we expressed our appreciation for her, and shared memories and the tangible impact she'd had on every one of us. But the most striking aspect to me was that everything she said suggested that she had done exactly as people aspire to: live lifed fully, with no regrets.

"I don't regret spending my life's work on research," she said. "My work mattered to me. And I want students to look at my life and think, *I can do something meaningful even in a short time.* I've had a very fulfilling life."

Tica struggled with the same daily challenges we all do: balancing work and family, the obligations of life in competition with our passions. But overall, she was able to look at her life and see that she'd lived her values and passions to the fullest extent that she could. I realized that I wanted to be able to say the same.

Recently, I received some amazing news: Tica's doctor was persistent in trying new drugs, and she is doing better! But living with a diagnosis like hers means constantly having to confront knowledge that the time to make any changes to how you spend your days is now. When she invited us all into her experience that day, she gave us a generous gift: the gentle prompt to look at our days and ask ourselves, from a big-picture perspective: *Am I living my best life? Where do I want to put my energy, and what can I let go of?*

Earlier I described how as we get older we feel more positive, and our social relationships are more positive. It's not about age though. It's about the perception of time: the less time we perceive we have left in life, the more we switch our goals toward more emotionally meaningful ones, including helping others.[11] In other words, when we think we have less time to live, we spend our time on what's truly meaningful to us. This can be called *spiritual urgency* and is a gift we can put in our go bag. Having spiritual urgency can give you a sense of freedom: Jump toward the more meaningful goals now. Live *now* as if it is your last year.

PRIORITIES INVENTORY

If you had only a year left to live, how would you want to spend your time?

Whom would you want to spend it with?

What would an ideal day look like?

Asking these questions helps us identify what we value. It helps us realize our priorities, align them with our day-to-day, and, when possible, get rid of things that don't align.

Earlier, I asked you to list all the stressors in your life. That might have included people who add stress to your life. Now, focus on people who enrich your life: Who makes you feel happy, loved, elevated? You might think about all the people who enrich your life, and how to make more time for them. Maybe you can try to see or talk to them more frequently, to start.

We might not be able to control how long we live, but we *can* adjust so that we're living more *now* as if it were our last year—so that we are living out our values and priorities. As we'll talk about later in this book, living a life that has meaning, and purpose, is one of the greatest ways to buffer stress.

Of course, some of those things that don't align may be nonnegotiable—there are plenty of responsibilities in life we can't opt out of, like certain tasks in our jobs, or caretaking. What do we do about the things we can't change?

The Things You Can't Change

Let's come back to Jane. She was in a situation that was particularly plagued with uncertainty (an uncertain medical future for her mother; an uncertain career future for herself) and was quite naturally trying to gain some degree of power over her circumstances. Everything had changed so suddenly. Sometimes, as Jane sat up late reading medical journals about neuroplasticity after stroke, she felt that if she just found the right set of information, she could roll back the clock and make her mother the way she was before. Meanwhile, things she *did* have a degree of influence over (like her job performance) were slipping through her fingers.

We spend a ton of mental energy attempting to solve things

that are beyond our control. Our distress lies in that friction between what we believe should be possible and what is possible. We can't control other people. We can't control whether a blood vessel contracts in somebody's brain. We can't control the past. In dialectical behavior therapy, one of the practices offered to people who are really struggling with extreme emotions and rumination (replaying over and over thoughts or situations that have already occurred) is to simply remind themselves: *This has happened. Reality is as it is.*[12] With some coaching, Jane started saying this to herself about her mother's illness: *This is happening. This is the reality.* Yes, she felt sad sometimes. But she also felt calmer. Less scattered and exhausted.

I'm so glad Jane was able to make this mental pivot. Because what we see with caregivers across multiple studies is that it's not the caregiving itself that accelerates cellular aging. It's secondary reactions from wanting the situation to be different than it is. Caregivers have more frequent thoughts of rejecting their present moment, which we call *negative mind wandering*: wishing you were somewhere else or doing something different.[13] These thoughts predict less happiness. We've found that it also affects your aging and is linked to shorter telomeres.[14]

Should you just passively accept every setback that life throws your way? No, I wouldn't recommend that! But you can work to improve the situation without trying to exert your will over factors that you can never really change. Jane was not going to change the course of her mother's illness, no matter how much googling she did, and there was no way to make sure that her mom would be 100 percent, absolutely safe at home alone. What she could do was ask her mother to wear a medical alert neck-lace. Her mother chafed at first, but Jane shopped around and found a pretty rose-gold necklace, shaped like a flower. She framed it as a favor: "I need to be able to focus at work, without worrying, and it would help me out if you'd wear it for me." Her mother put the necklace on.

Shortly after, Jane was able to move out into her own place nearby. Things at work got quickly better, as she had more men-tal bandwidth to devote to it. It was hard not to spend time wishing things were different—she did find herself whirring on what-ifs from time to time. *What if I had noticed the symptoms? What if they had caught it faster?* But most of the time, she was able to catch herself slipping into that ruminative pattern and pull back.

When I catch myself trying to change something that's not within my control, I take a moment and visualize it as though I'm pulling on a rope that's tied to something immovable, like an enormous boulder. I'm using up all my energy trying to solve something that cannot be solved. That rock will never budge. I gently ask myself: *Can I just drop the rope and let it be?*[15] Or some-times, for a particularly sticky situation that is hard to walk away from, it takes an emphatic *"Drop the rope!"* and some rad-ical acceptance, which we will practice next.

Acceptance and Finding Peace within Pain

When we can't control a situation, we can still control how we respond to it. Many turn to mindfulness meditation here because it focuses a lot on acceptance of feelings and thoughts. In one study, researchers compared the efficacy of two different mindfulness classes, which guided participants through short daily meditations.[16] The first group used an app that encouraged focused attention along with awareness of their attention: so, placing focus on the breath, and then moving it back to the breath whenever they became aware that it had wandered. (Many studies have found that this practice is beneficial for focus and attention—especially the *awareness* piece, which is what allows you to notice when you begin mind wandering or ruminating.) The second group used a different app, one that added *acceptance* of one's state—not just awareness of thoughts and feelings, but kind acceptance of them, especially of negative experiences that we typically push away. Both groups had attentional benefits. But only the second group—the *acceptance* group—had an improved *stress reactivity profile*, which is our capacity to respond to and recover from events in a healthy way, and more positive emotions to boot.[17] *Acceptance* was the piece that actually led to stress resilience.

Most of us know that when you're caught in a riptide, the advice is always the same: *Don't fight it.* Don't argue with reality. You will exhaust yourself and only get pulled farther out to sea. Riptides are simply too strong—we're no match for them. The only way to stay afloat is to swim *with* the current, surf the tide. Go with it; see where it takes you. Maybe you can leverage it in a different way. There are creative ways of working with strong negative emotions to grow, rather than avoiding them—

more guidance on this is described in "Further Reading and Resources."

Radical acceptance is, at a basic level, accepting that something terrible or traumatic happened. It's a mental stance that embraces the reality that we cannot change the event, and that radical acceptance is a better option than the alternative: avoiding, rejecting reality, fighting the riptide, and feeling victimized (*Why me?*). It can decrease painful emotions of shame, guilt, sadness, and anger about the event. This has been a helpful method for people with excessive emotional swings, PTSD, and chronic pain.[18] Radical acceptance is what helped Jane accept her mother's condition and her new life as a caregiver.

There are so many things that have happened or will happen to us in life that we did not ask for, did not want, and that are tremendously disappointing and painful and take a lot of time and work to adjust to. Most are uncontrollable events or situations. These are opportunities for building strength and resilience, even though we didn't ask to build it. These low points become the foundation for growth: when you have no other options, you find strength you didn't know you had. This takes both acceptance and managing our expectations and emotions around it. You are going to start practicing radical acceptance today—but know it usually isn't an overnight or onetime thing. It's an iterative process. Once we feel the pain coming on about a situation, we can make a U-turn and try radical acceptance of the situation, and acceptance about our emotional responses as well.

Of course, not everything can be sorted cleanly into "what I can control" and "what I can't control." There are degrees and gray areas. We always need to be evaluating where to put our cognitive and emotional energy, assessing when to push through a tough spot and when to release and ride the current.

On Day 1, we talked about identifying unconscious tension caused by the inherent uncertainty of life and letting it go. We practiced "catch and release"—training ourselves to *notice* when we're holding the stress of uncertainty and releasing it. Today, we go one step further and look outward, noticing the specific conditions of our lives that are keeping us in a stressed state.

TODAY'S PRACTICE

CONTROL WHAT YOU CAN . . . AND PUT DOWN THE REST

Go-Bag Skill: Letting Go When It No Longer Serves You

Take Stock

Make a list of all the stressful situations in your life using the Stress Inventory on page 35. If you already did this as you were reading the chapter, great—go right to the next step. If not, flip back and make your list now. Nothing is too small or specific for this list. For big issues (like work, parenting challenges, relationship problems), try to write down specific situations, whatever really stresses you out.

Delete What You Can

Look at your list and cross out any situations that you can exit or end. For example: If there is a project that you don't have time for, or that is causing too much strife, what if you were to drop that goal, or delegate that project? Visualize your day *minus* that particular stressor.

If nothing jumps out as an easy delete, answer these questions: If you were *forced* to drop one thing, what would it be? What could you (and others) live without? What would you lose? What would be the worst thing about dropping it? And how does that negative compare with the consequences of keeping it? (See the "Can I Push the Delete Button?" section earlier in this chapter.) Most of us don't feel we have enough time in our day, so pruning things, simplifying our day, and focusing on our priority list not only reduces stress, but can create more room for ease and spaciousness, and for adding things that bring you joy and purpose.

Are you ready to try?

If your honest answer is no, that's okay. We'll come back to this at the end of the book, in "Renewing Your Prescription."

But if you can, dump something today. See how it feels to take one thing off your plate—even if it is small.

Establish Your Sphere of Influence: A Circle for Control

Now look at your list and circle any situations that you sense you can influence or improve. This is where you can focus some of your mental energy today. Write next to each circle one small thing you can do to start improving the situation. For instance, you might find the morning rush is stressful. This is actually one of the most common times of the day people regularly feel stressed. Can you consider tweaking your sleep or wake-up time, or planning your clothes, meals, and daily schedule the night before? For some issues (financial strain, parenting, work), you can't change things alone, and so there might be initial conversations you can have with others to start the process of small changes. Work stress is common and can be broken down into aspects you can control and cannot control. Is there a supervisor at work who is treating you poorly? This is a tough situation but one worth problem-solving, maybe with a friend. In extreme cases, changing a toxic work situation may mean needing to find a different job.

Know What You Need to Accept: A Box for the Bricks

Looking again at your list, draw a box around the situations or stressors that you have zero (or very little) control over. Examples: A loved one's illness or addiction. A project you cannot get rid of. The possibility that you will be stuck inside for days or weeks due to extreme weather. A traumatic event.

Allow some control. For each of these stressors, ask yourself: *Is there anything within this scenario that I have control over that would help, and reduce feelings of powerlessness?* For example, Jane couldn't control whether her mother might fall again, but she could buy her a medical alert necklace. I can't control when the next major fire near my home will happen; it's just a matter of time. But I now have enough air purifiers (and a go bag!). Most situations are not completely uncontrollable, because they can be navigated with more ease. If there's a simple task you can do that will put you in the driver's seat (even as you accept that you don't control the bends in the road that are coming!), then add it to your to-do list for later in the week.

Allow self-compassion. For some of the boxed items, you'll need to take a different approach: acceptance and self-compassion. One thing you can do for situations you cannot change is to acknowledge how hard this is; to welcome in your feelings about it rather than push them away. Can you identify any feelings of pain (such as sadness, rejection, anger, resentment), and let them be? They are valid; they are natural responses. What would you say to comfort a close friend in this situation? Can you show this kindness to yourself?

Finally, drop the luggage! Picture each box as a heavy brick in a suitcase you're carrying around. It exists; it's not going anywhere. But you don't need to carry it around with you. You can set your luggage down for a while. Stories of pain are especially heavy; check if you are carrying any bricks made of those. If it helps, draw a little handle on the tops of all of those boxes containing stressful situations outside your control. Now, before you progress to the next part of your day, visualize yourself setting those bricks down in a safe place, just for a while. Don't think about whether it's realistic or possible to never worry about this problem again—it will come up again. But if you're carrying this stress with you *all the time*, you're going to be exhausted and worn out. Your health is going to suffer. And you're going to be less capable of meeting other challenges when they come along. For now, drop the baggage! You don't have to carry these bricks around all day.

Bonus Practice

For the tough things you cannot change, consider practicing radical acceptance. This means accepting the situation completely: in your mind, your heart, and your body. This is hard to do. That's why it's a *practice*: something you do over and over again until it sinks in. It's when we stop ignoring, fighting, or trying to alter reality that we can actually feel calmness, with all of the physiological benefits it brings. Accepting it does not mean you approve of it. Instead, you are choosing not to make yourself more miserable by fighting it.

To practice radical acceptance, try this exercise:

Think of a situation that bothers you deeply that has already happened, or that cannot be changed, and that you find hard to accept.

1. Close your eyes and focus on your breath.
2. Scan for painful thoughts about the situation that may arise, such as: *The situation isn't fair* or *I can't live with this* or *Why me?*
3. Meet the painful thought with a statement of acceptance and certainty, such as: *It is what it is* or *This is reality* or *It happened* or *Things are exactly as they are right now.*

4. Allow and acknowledge sadness, grief, disappointment. Notice sensations in the body.

5. Put your hands on your chest, with kindness, and spread feelings of warmth and kindness through your body. Remind yourself, with a long, slow exhale: *I can gently put this baggage down right now.* Repeat that until you feel lighter.

Troubleshooting

Sometimes it's hard to come up with the specific things that are weighing on us. Our sources of stress can be vague, undefined, or obscured . . . or we can be totally off base. We think it's one thing that's causing our stress to skyrocket (*all those dishes in the sink!*) when it's really something else completely (tension in a relationship, financial strain, career unhappiness, etc.), or it's ten little things. If you had trouble filling out your Stress Inventory, try this method that helps identify worries. This practice also helps people who worry too much contain their worry to a limited window of time.

The Worry Window

Get several pieces of paper and something to write with, a computer or tablet to type on, or a recorder to talk into, and set a timer on your phone for five minutes. When you push the start button, you have only one job: to worry.

You are creating a worry window now.

We spend a lot of time trying to rein in the mind when it

starts to worry about things that haven't happened and may never happen . . . and that cognitive wrestling takes a toll. So right now, for the next five minutes, let your mind be free, and go to the hot zones. Let it worry about whatever it wants to worry about. Let it indulge in catastrophizing to its heart's content. Don't censor yourself—write down as many worries as come to you. Big or small, catch it on paper so you can look at it more objectively, naming it, deciding if you want to worry more about it. What's the situation behind the worry? If you cannot identify the source of the anxiety, name qualities of the anxiety—size, shape, temperature, color. Defining it helps you work with it.

You might see that many of these worries are really just intolerance of uncertainty, things unlikely to happen, as we talked about in Day 1. You might visualize these low-probability situations flying out the window. Then focus on the big stressful situations in front of you—identify what you can change right now and what you can't.

Paradoxically, it turns out that setting a time to worry reduces worry for the rest of the day. You may very well end with a sense of having "gotten it out of your system" for the day. You put your worries all on paper, so you don't need to keep them circulating in your mind. You contained them. And you get to worry in this contained way again tomorrow! Set an alert on your phone to do a worry window at roughly the same time tomorrow. If worries pop up later today, remind yourself that you have time set aside for that worrying tomorrow. If you often have trouble pinning down what's stressing you out, or feel the general vagueness and tension of uncertainty, the worry window might be a great routine for you.

You Might Want a Worry Window for Two!

A worry window for two works if the stressful situation you have is with a family member or partner you live with. When there is conflict with someone you live with, home can be a stressful place. But because our home is where we sleep and eat, it's important to put a container on the conflict, keep it in a box that you control together. Limit the amount of time you talk and think about this conflict. You might consider setting aside fifteen minutes for a worry window discussion. Remember that really seeing the other's views and validating feelings can be helpful, and that peace is often better than being right. My partner and I had been dealing with an ongoing, seemingly unsolvable situation that we held different views about, and therapy didn't help. We planned a time each week to really listen, share our views, and talk about next steps—and then when the time was up, we stopped. We tried not to bring the subject up until our next "teatime" (worry window) talk.

DAY 3

BE THE LION

PICTURE A LION HUNTING A GAZELLE, MERCILESSLY RUNNING HER down across the hot savannah. The gazelle is terrified and in fight-or-flight mode, sprinting for her life. The lion is exhilarated, anticipating her hard-fought meal as she closes the gap. Which animal is experiencing stress—the lion or the gazelle?

The answer is *both*.

Both nervous systems are highly activated and undergoing physiological changes they can't control. Yet they're experiencing stress arousal in two very different ways. The gazelle is locked in a threat response. She is full of fear, coursing with adrenaline. Her blood flow is constricted because her vessels have narrowed (*vasoconstriction*) to prevent excessive bleeding. Less oxygen makes it to the brain as physiological resources are directed to the limbs. Her body has become a machine with only one purpose: outrun the predator. Meanwhile, the lion is having a challenge response. Her heart is pumping volumes of blood efficiently, allowing her maximal speed and anticipating the meal she's about to have. She is focused and driven. She seems to have unlimited reserves of energy.

These are two very different physiological profiles, but *stress* is the constant. The difference is how each player responds to stress—how they perceive it, and therefore how they experience it, mentally and physically. The difference between the lion and the gazelle? The gazelle perceived a threat: her life was in danger. The lion perceived a challenge: her next meal.

Of course, I'm not suggesting that in a real-life scenario, a gazelle can simply change her perspective—she'll get eaten! But in this clear-cut example from the animal world, there is a lesson here for us. Most of us are not regularly being chased by life-threatening lions. But our bodies are behaving as though we are. Too often, we're responding to the stressors that pop up over the course of a day as though they're a survival threat to fight off or run from, rather than a meal to take down. Our bodies shoot into fight-or-flight mode, dumping cortisol and adrenaline into our bloodstreams, rocketing our nervous systems into a state of fear and vigilance. And when that response happens, full blown or even half blown, with each stressful or unexpected event that comes along, our bodies no longer know how to "come down" from the stress.

Are You More Lion, or More Gazelle?

We all respond to stress so differently from each other. Why do some people stew in the soup of stress daily, overreacting to small things, while others let big, threatening events bounce off them as if they had a shield around them?

Part of studying stress means digging into the universal ways that the human brain works; on the other hand, we also have to look at how unique each person is. We each have a highly personal lens through which we see the world, shaped by our genetics and personal life experiences, and by little changes in our day, like how much sleep we had the night before and what we ate. Events unfold, and we perceive them in a certain way, through our own mental filter.[1]

Why might we each respond differently to similar events? Well, the brain is constantly processing sensory input from our body and environment, and comparing that input with our memories of the past in order to best predict the future. The human brain is a predictive machine; it uses our personal past as data. Even our early childhood experiences will shape how we respond to little things. People who suffered from a lot of early life adversity often develop mind habits that keep them in yellow mind: they feel heightened baseline levels of daily stress, whether or not a stressful event happens. They feel a greater sense that their lives are threatened by stressful events—it doesn't take much to push them into a catastrophic red mind stress response.

We have more of a "predicting brain" than a "reality brain." That means we may be responding to something we predict or believe will happen, rather than what *is* happening. (As Michel de Montaigne said, "There were many terrible events in my life, and most of them never happened.") But there is a way to inter-vene in this process.

Dr. Stefanie Mayer of UCSF found that people with early childhood trauma have exaggerated threat appraisals of their daily stressors, which contribute to later depression.[2] In her fol-lowing study on a similar group, she pinged them during the day to invite them to have a moment of mindful awareness of their thoughts, and feelings of self-compassion. She found that after a brief mindful check-in, they had more "challenge appraisals," meaning they felt they could cope better with their daily events, and had more positive emotions.[3] In other words, when we can shift the way we *perceive* daily stressors to view them as less threatening, we change our stress response. We can feel more like a lion than a gazelle.

Getting out of Gazelle Mode

Steven had worked for Kodak for his entire career, handling major accounts with large retailers like Target and Walmart. Then the bottom fell out of the film industry. The shift to dig-ital had been coming for a while, but when the stock market crashed in 2008, many film companies radically downsized in an attempt to stay in the game. And Steven was part of that downsizing. At sixty, he found it tough to start over in a new career—a lot of avenues he tried turned out to be dead ends. Fi-nally he decided to do something he'd always wanted to do: run for office.

He'd thought about going into politics for a long time, but it never seemed to be the right time to leave a stable career. But now, the current mayor of his small New England town had announced that she wouldn't be seeking another term. It seemed like a good time to go for it.

He knew it would be stressful. He just didn't know *how* stressful. The run-up to the election itself became contentious—his opponent wasn't afraid to go dirty, and did so at every turn. He couldn't pick up the local paper or check Facebook without wondering if there'd be some new attack against him. He was constantly tense, scanning, alert. He told himself that it was just the election season—it would be over soon. But then, a twist: he won the election.

What had seemed like "just a couple of months" had morphed into a four-year term. Now, the stressors all appeared at his office door, in the form of citizens with various complaints and problems. The phone rang all day. There were emergencies. Budget issues. If he made any kind of mistake, critics swarmed. The many questions constituents asked that he couldn't immediately answer sent a stab of panic through him as he scrambled to figure out a response. Steven would get stuck thinking about all the ways he could have done things differently. He started to worry: *Maybe I'm not cut out for this job.*

If a medical professional were to have stepped into his office in the middle of all this to check his vitals, they would have found shallow breathing, an elevated heart rate, and higher than usual levels of cortisol in the blood. This was not sustainable for a four-year term—and he knew it. He just didn't know what to do about it.

Because unmanaged chronic stress wears down telomeres and hastens cell senescence, it can usher us too early into the "disease-span": the period in our lives when we start to develop the illnesses of aging. Chronic stress shifts our behavior and appetite. It drives us toward comfort foods (those with high sugar and fat). Believing it needs to conserve resources for survival, the body slows metabolism and stores fat in the inner abdominal area. High stress arousal keeps us from sleeping well, so we're constantly depleted. It drives addiction. "Stress brain" turns on brain pathways that crave pleasure and relief, making calorie-dense foods more rewarding and driving insulin resistance, inflammation, and obesity.

At the same time, our acute stress response—the short-term response we turn on when under pressure—is an amazing capacity we have. Our bodies are built to handle that type of transient stress. When something negative or challenging happens, or when we anticipate that it will, we mount this beautiful, sharp, peak response. In the blink of an eye, blood pressure goes up, the nervous system becomes more vigilant, and cortisol and adrenaline, the primary stress hormones, are reflexively released into the bloodstream. The sympathetic nervous system (fight or flight) turns the volume to high while the parasympathetic (rest and digest) turns down, allowing us to have this intense, energizing stress response. This fast, powerful biological domino effect helps us focus on danger, have more energy, and react quickly. Our acute stress response is a huge asset—we would never want to be without it. But we need a "quick shutoff." We need that stress response to *end* when the stress-inducing incident does.

Let's pause here for some good news: you've already been working on this. The techniques we practiced in the first two chapters were designed to help us regulate our stress response better. When we can expect the unexpected and remain mentally open and flexible to a range of possibilities, it takes the teeth out of unanticipated issues that crop up—you don't have that knee-jerk "gazelle" response. And when we have a clear idea of what we can and can't control, we're less likely to spend our time planning for the unplannable. Both of these strategies are going to help you shift toward a healthier, more balanced stress experience. But there's a critical next step: being able to see daily stressful events as challenges, not threats. And that's easier said than done.

It's one thing to understand that you "should" approach sudden, upsetting, or stressful situations in your life as challenges rather than threats; it's another to make that mental shift in the moment, as things unfold. But there are some specific strategies we can use to do exactly that. And the first is to start thinking about our stress response as an asset so we don't feel threatened by stress itself.

Your Stress Is Your Strength

To study the difference between *threat stress* and *challenge stress*, my colleague Wendy Mendes manipulates people's stress responses in the lab. She gives them situations they can rise up to and feel control over, versus creating really uncomfortable, novel situations that induce threat responses both emotionally and physiologically. She's found that the more we feel in control and equipped with resources—what we call a *challenge mindset*—the more we have a positive stress response. Challenge responses are characterized by feeling more positive emotion, and by more blood pumping from the heart (cardiac output), instead of the vasoconstriction (narrowing of the blood vessels) that we experience with a threat response. Feeling more challenge than threat before a stressor is even related to longer telomeres, which as we know is linked to longevity and vitality.[4]

Many of us feel threatened by the stress response itself. But the science shows that with some practice, we *can* manipulate our own stress response. Teaching people to view their stress response as a strength leads to a challenge mindset and physiology, and better coping.[5] Accomplishing this may be as simple as *telling ourselves* that our stress response is helping us.

In one classic study, Mendes and her colleagues taught students to view their stress response as helping them do well on an important exam, and their performance actually went up—the opposite of test anxiety![6] Dr. Alia Crum, a researcher at Stanford, developed a Stress Mindset Measure to help people assess their beliefs about stress.[7]

YOUR STRESS MINDSET

How much do you believe each statement, on a scale of 1 (not at all) to 10 (extremely)? Think about stressful events, not chronic toxic stress.

STRESS IS HARMFUL	Rating (1–10)	STRESS IS HELPFUL	Rating (1–10)
Stress should be completely avoided		Stress should be sought and utilized	
Stress inhibits my learning and growth		Stress enhances my learning and growth	
Stress depletes my health and vitality		Stress improves my health and vitality	
Total score:		**Total score:**	

Dr. Crum found that our stress mindset is malleable: If you present people with information about the harmful effects of stress, they do worse. If you tell them the benefits of stress, they tend to do better. It's that simple. When we focus on the benefits of stress, we feel less stress about stress, pay attention to positive cues rather than threatening cues, and approach situations more confidently rather than avoid them. With positive stress beliefs, people feel more engaged in their work, more positive emotions, and less physiological reactivity. What you're telling yourself matters! If you scored high on the harmful side in the

set Measure, you might focus your attention more
ts of stress, and remind yourself of these right be-
...re you deal with some thorny situation.

So first and foremost, when you feel your stress response starting up—a surge of alarm, racing heart, damp palms, high energy, or jitteriness—remember that the capacity to mount a stress response to a difficult situation is a strength, not a weakness. Think of it this way: asking for support when you are struggling is a strength (which we heard a lot during the pandemic); this is your body asking for the help it needs in that stressful moment so it can be stronger. For Steven, this reframe helped enormously—when he started to think of his stress response as something that was designed to help him tackle the challenges of his new role, the moments of high stress just didn't feel as toxic. He was even able to welcome it (*Okay, bring it on! Energize me!*), and he recovered more quickly afterward.

Your body is built to recover from stress quickly. The human nervous system can go back to baseline within minutes, and most hormones return to normal levels within half an hour (the inflammatory cytokines stick around a bit longer, in case they are needed for wound healing). That's the gold standard of a healthy stress response: quickly rebounding from acute stress. You have this capacity already—you just need to get out of your own way and let your body do what it's programmed to do. And it's a lot easier for our bodies to "come down" in a timely and healthy way after a *challenge* experience instead of a *threat* experience. The biological and mental residue of a threat experience sticks around—we ruminate and relive. Challenges are different—like scaling a mountain, we hit the peak and then come down the other side.

I want you to hold these two important points in mind as we progress through the rest of this week:

My stress response is an asset—it helps me rise to the challenge.
I can recover quickly from stress—my body was built to do it.

This understanding of human biology—that stress is not inherently unhealthy or to be avoided, and that your natural stress response is not "wrong"—is a critical foundation for flipping from a threat response to a challenge response. For Steven, it helped him to be less reactive about the stress he was experiencing and the way he was responding. When he understood the utility of it, he was less self-critical and more accepting. But he needed to do more. Election season was one thing—a few months of high stress won't damage anyone irreparably; the body has a great capacity to recover from stress. But a four-year term—or longer—was a concern. The stressors of this job weren't going anywhere, so for this career to be sustainable for his health, he was going to have to learn how to respond to them differently. But how do you make that switch?

Take the Threat out of Stress

A big part of Steven's challenge was that he was in a new and unfamiliar role. Any one of us can slip into this threat response mode when we feel pushed back on our heels, faced with the unknown. A disappointing outcome for a work initiative, a less-than-rosy moment in your parenting life, a fight with someone important to you—all of these, and more, can set us off into feeling that we've failed, or are failing, in some fundamental way.

The first reframe we have to make is realizing that failure is part of success. It may seem like the easier path is to avoid new situations, to minimize risk and avoid pain. Anytime you are pursuing something worth going after—a career in the sciences, a new role in politics, trying to launch a business, becoming a new parent—mistakes will inevitably be a large part of that journey. Making mistakes is common, generic, part of our growth path. *Expect* failure as normal, not catastrophic and not personal to you. We know that successful people take risks—they put themselves out there and vulnerable to experiencing multiple failures. The only true failure is giving up on something that takes persistence. Knowing that mistakes and failure are simply part of the process of achieving goals helps us have less of a threat response, more of a challenge response.

THREAT STRESS BELIEF:

If I fail, it means I'm not cut out for this.

REFRAME:

If I fail, it means I'm challenging myself.

Steven realized that in politics, failure was the rule, not the exception (as in business, as in the arts, as in discovery science, and so on). Most of the initiatives he took up were not going to progress—there was political opposition, budgeting restraints, voter referendums that would determine what actually got done. For every success he had in office, he would experience ten times that many failures—and that was part of being an effective town leader. His failures were a sign he was working toward something worthwhile. With that reframe, he didn't feel threatened by failures anymore. He was able to experience stress more as a driver and motivator and less as a predator breathing down his neck. No more gazelling!

THREAT STRESS BELIEF:

I'll never be able to pull this off.

REFRAME:

I have what it takes to figure this out.

And if I struggle, I can ask for help.

One reason you may feel sharp pangs in performance situations is that your self-talk tells you things that are quite the opposite of the helpful thoughts of a challenge mindset: that you are not good enough, you don't deserve your credentials, you don't belong, you're not up to par. In the extreme case, this becomes *impostor syndrome*: you fear being discovered as a fraud. This can really derail you. It can prevent you from setting personal career goals. Impostorism is strongly related to low self-esteem, self-doubt, and a lack of self-compassion, and puts you at risk of underachievement and burnout.[8] It can lead to both fear of failure and fear of success.[9]

And the funny thing about impostorism is that it doesn't even matter how much evidence you have that you're actually succeeding: It is common in high achievers, even in people at the highest level of their profession. Around 30 percent or more of medical students, surgery residents, and attendings have the syndrome.[10]

Impostor syndrome fuels the threat mindset. It feels like being on shaky ground—when what's foremost in your mind are all the reasons you aren't skilled enough, experienced enough, *whatever* enough to succeed, it's pretty impossible to feel like a lion.

Self-talk is a simple yet superpowerful tool in our go bag: how we talk to ourselves can either amplify our stress or bring us directly to a calmer state.

Most of us have had the thought *I don't deserve this, I shouldn't be here, I'm not as good at this as I should be.* This self-talk sounds the same whether you're talking about a job or a scholastic or personal achievement. To counter this false but common self-sabotage, turn your attention to your internal compass: judge yourself compared with your past performance, not based on others' performances or expectations, and not based on overly rigid or perfectionistic standards.

Even though Steven was new to politics, he *did* have the skills and competencies that he needed to be successful in that role. He finally let go of that inner chatter telling him he was going to be revealed as an imposter. He'd been fixated on all the industry knowledge he'd relied on in his previous role, and which he lacked in this one. However, Steven had developed other critical skills that made him uniquely suited to the role of mayor that he just hadn't been focusing on: he was good at finding common ground, a fast learner, a clear communicator, and an innovative problem solver. When he pulled these vital skills to the front of his mind leading up to a tough conversation, public debate, or other high-stress task, and reminded himself of the other times he'd succeeded in a similar situation, he felt less flappable.

THREAT STRESS BELIEF:

If I don't pull this off, everything will be ruined.

REFRAME:

I can only do my best; everything else is out of my control.

Researchers have tested the effects of a perspective shift called *spontaneous self-distancing.* In many studies, it tamps down anxious and emotional reactivity to future stressors.[11] What does "self-distancing" mean? It means that when some people feel stress about something coming up, they *zoom outward*. They look at the situation from a "self-distanced" perspective, rather than a "self-immersed" perspective. They take in the bigger picture, and their bodies respond more calmly to the stressor. The lesson: if you can "unhook" yourself from the important task you are doing and remember what about it is important and to whom, you can feel more positive challenge and less toxic threat.

One of the best ways to achieve healthy psychological distancing is by putting some time between yourself and this stressful event. No, you can't time travel, of course, but you can do so in your mind.

Zoom into the future and ask yourself: *In the longer term, how much will this thing matter? How much will it affect me in a week? A month? A year? A decade?*

It's funny—sometimes if I'm venting about a situation at the dinner table, my son has learned to throw one of my own questions right back at me. "Mom," he says, "how much will this matter in five years?"

It's always a great reset. It shrinks the importance of the situation. It's still there, it just doesn't take up as much space in my mind or in my life. When stressors grow so big that they start to fill your whole lens, it's time to do a perspective check. Often, upcoming stressful events will have gained a size and weight in our minds that they just don't deserve. We all have just one life to live. We can feel more *challenged* rather than *threatened* by keeping a healthy perspective.

THREAT STRESS BELIEF:

This is so stressful. I hate this feeling.

REFRAME:

This is exciting! I can appreciate this feeling!

This might seem too simple to be real. But simply telling your-self that something is exciting, rather than threatening, can help shift you toward a positive stress experience. Saying things to change your view about stress, or making *reappraisal state-ments*, has been tested in thirty-six studies now.[12] While these statements sometimes improve your autonomic nervous system responses, they reliably reduce your emotional stress. In other words, your beliefs about stress can take a huge bite of out of the negative stress you feel and empower you to perform better.

This can look like viewing stress itself as life enhancing (a positive stress mindset), viewing your physical stress response as performance enhancing (*My sweaty palms and elevated heart rate are helping me—my body is excited!*), or viewing yourself as empowered and prepared instead of threatened. If you are able to put in time, a regular mindfulness practice can help you flip that stress response from *threat* to *challenge*: in a study we ran at UCSF, we found that mindfulness training allowed partici-pants to maintain higher levels of positive "challenge" emotions (such as feelings of excitement and confidence) after a stressor, and that they had greater cardiac output and less vasoconstric-tion.[13] Mindfulness teaches metacognition—the ability to ob-serve our minds—so it makes it easier to adopt reframes.

So know this: To a certain extent, you can shape your own

nse! You might feel the spike of adrenaline at work,
ou *can choose* how to interpret your body's natural
onse and improve how things unfold.

Until Steven sat down to think through these threat-to-challenge reframes, he didn't even realize that a lot of his threat stress was coming from one big problem: he'd taken office with an impossible goal. *Making everyone happy*. He was used to doing that in the marketing world, where the goal was happy customers. Running a town was an entirely different beast. He needed to radically reframe his idea of success: if he did one thing to make the town better in his four years in office, he decided, he was going to consider it a win.

In the end, there were more failures than wins over the four years, and yes, they were often stressful. But he had adopted a positive stress mindset and viewed the challenges as the path to success, a necessary bridge to cross on the road to the things he *did* accomplish, which then allowed him to react to them differently. For the most part, Steven was able to feel motivated, driven, and energized by the job—not perpetually stressed, attacked, and depleted. And when he did find himself skewing too far over into the threatened "red mind" zone, he could use these mental reframes to get himself back on track.

After four years (even though he didn't make everyone happy) Steven was reelected. In his second term, he faced a new stress resilience task: to not overidentify with the role of "mayor." This is the final, and arguably the hardest, mental pivot to make as we seek to become the lion: to not tie our identity and self-worth to one particular role or facet of our lives.

Don't Put All Your Eggs in One Basket

If you're a basketball fan, you might be familiar with Kevin Love, power forward for the Cleveland Cavaliers. Love is a highly accomplished athlete: he's a five-time NBA All-Star, has been to the Olympics, and won an NBA championship with the Cavaliers in 2016. He's also the son of an NBA player. He's been recognized for his achievements in the sport for almost his entire life. I had the honor of having a dialogue with him on a radio event presented by the Commonwealth Club, and learned about his experience with impostorism and "identity threat stress."[14] It started with a cry for help from his nervous system.

In 2017, during a home game against the Atlanta Hawks, Love suffered a panic attack. In an essay he shared a few months after the incident, he described a perfect storm of stress and pressure leading up to the game: interpersonal issues with his family, trouble sleeping, and high expectations for his performance in the game that he feared he couldn't meet.[15] His struggle began as soon as the game did. He felt exhausted and winded. His game was off—he kept missing baskets—and he felt like his brain was spinning. Finally, he left the court with a racing heart and ended up at the hospital, getting a battery of tests. He was fine. But at the next game, the same thing happened.

Love started therapy after his panic attacks, and realized that a big part of the immense stress he was experiencing was due to how tightly yoked his identity was to his profession and his performance. He shared his own experience with the hope that it would help other athletes—or anyone whose self-worth is strongly shaped by their performance in one particular arena of their lives. His point was that if you identify as a "great basketball player" and have a bad game, you're devastated. It's hard to recover from. He wrote, "When I wasn't performing, I didn't feel like I was succeeding as a person."

When we feel our personhood is under attack, we are in gazelle mode. So if you're in gazelle mode and aren't sure why, take a moment and ask yourself: *What about this situation is making my sense of self feel threatened?* When your core identity is threatened, and you have "all your eggs in one basket," this is a recipe for feeling threatened. Maybe what you find most valuable about yourself (or believe that others find valuable about you) is your ability to be a good parent. Maybe it's your capacity to be a high earner. Maybe it's that you always produce great results on deadline. Whatever it is, you may find that the normal bumps and snags that occur in these roles affect you more strongly and more frequently. When "who you are" is on the line, your "status" is threatened, and your body will respond as though it's being attacked.

There's a cultural message we receive that shapes our values unconsciously, which is that we have to achieve, acquire, and perform exceptionally to have value. It leads to us feeling low self-worth with any setback—especially when it's tied to one outcome (hit this deadline, make this sale, publish this study . . . fill in the blank!). The solution?

Diversify.

I don't mean *do* more. Instead, remember all the other things you already are. None of us are just one thing. As Love put it, "What you do for a living doesn't have to define who you are."

Remind yourself of the things you care about, and the other roles you play in life, besides the one at stake. As Steven worked through his second and then third terms as mayor, this was how he pulled himself back from a chronic stress cycle. So many people attached his identity to "mayor." It felt like that was why they valued and respected him. When he saw himself that way, the prospect of losing that title was devastating. So when big challenges came up at work—ones that might influence future elections—Steven managed his own stress by reminding himself of everything else he was. He was a wonderful father and a loving husband. He was an active community member, contributing to several boards and volunteer organizations. He was a dedicated son who managed his elderly parents' healthcare and finances. His identity—and his value to the world at a large—had many facets. It could not be reduced to just one role.

A powerful tactic here is to use *values affirmations* to reorient yourself to your inner compass and remember everything you *already do*. Some people feel that self-affirmations—positive statements about yourself—are corny and pointless, and feel self-conscious doing it. I get it—affirmations remind me of Stuart Smalley, a character from a famous *Saturday Night Live* comedy skit who would say each week, "I'm good enough, I'm smart enough, and doggone it, people like me!" But this isn't the kind of affirmation I'm talking about. The science shows that rmations—where you write down the core, driving your life, and then list all the ways you are currently living and embodying those values—are quite powerful. These are much more effective than general positive statements about ourselves (sorry, Stuart!). When we feel our personal integrity and ego are threatened, we can blunt the stress by reminding ourselves of our core values and any ways we are already working toward what we most care about.[16]

The research on this is exciting: values affirmations help improve students' grades, especially for Black and Hispanic students, and even increase medical residents' performance.[17] They can blunt stress hormones, such as cortisol and catecholamines. David Creswell, PhD, a researcher from Carnegie Mellon University, tested the role of affirmation: Women with breast cancer wrote about coping with cancer, once a week for three weeks, and their essays were analyzed for self-affirmations. For example, their affirmation could be "I prayed more than I ever have. Prayer has always been a personal strength of mine." Those who wrote more self-affirming statements had better health three months later.[18] He then wanted to test if affirmations can be "seen" in brain activity, and found that value affirmations activate the brain's reward areas (ventromedial prefrontal cortex), just like thinking about sex or happy memories. With repeated practice, thinking this way inoculates you against the threat response.[19]

Try this now! Choose a few strong values or personal strengths, possibly from the following list, and really think about why each matters to you and how you embody it.

MY CORE VALUES

Choose three values in your life (ideas below) and think of an example of how you are living them:

- Creativity/artistic/musical
- Community/relationships
- Being a good friend or family member
- Gaining knowledge / curiosity
- Helping others / social justice / equity
- Honesty / integrity / moral principles
- Courage/bravery
- Kindness/generosity/compassion
- Nature/environment/sustainability
- Spirituality/religion

With a solid foundation of where your worth and value really come from, you are much more able to physiologically mount a challenge response to stress, and to then recover from stress more quickly. This ability to see yourself with a multifaceted identity is a huge ingredient in stress resilience: with this self-knowledge, something threatening one part of your life can no longer threaten your whole being so completely.

When I lead stress management retreats, we coach people through this issue of "identity diversity"—of really expanding your sense of self to include everything you are. We don't want our self-worth to hinge on one small sliver of the pie—we want to see the whole pie, every day.

And it's not just about what you *do* and value—just being yourself is enough. Although we get messages from society that we are only as good as our achievements, we must remember and trust that our natural, inherent worth is always present, and that we have an expansive identity if we remind ourselves of it. At our retreats, we offer participants a mantra to fall back on: *I am enough.* Say it to yourself in moments when an issue in one arena of your life seems like an attack, a violation, a threat. Wrapped up in that short phrase is the knowledge that you are many things, and inherently worthy and important—no matter what happens.

I am enough, I have enough, and I do enough.

Given the implicit and explicit sexism we encounter over the course of our lives, women in particular develop more negative self-views, appraise stress more harshly, and just have higher average stress levels, in every study I have ever seen. Every person with a marginalized social identity faces this same challenge, in that they may have internalized stigma and hurtful messages. So it's especially important for us to examine what we are saying to ourselves. The self-critic's voice can be so loud and frequent that you no longer even notice it—you've accepted it. Tina Fey, the comedian who started out in improv clubs and then rose to fame on *Saturday Night Live*, has made me laugh so many times. Here's something she said that really gets me: "I am constantly amazed by Tina Fey. And I *am* Tina Fey."

I ask everyone in the retreat audience to repeat this using

their own name. It's super uncomfortable at first, but try it. Each one of you has survived countless hardships, losses, and rejections over your life, and yet you are still here, trying your best, trying to do better. Say it again. How much do you really believe it?

A participant in one of my workshops, Cathy Caplener, once said (half jokingly, I thought) that she was going to put up a big billboard with huge block letters that would say YOU ARE ENOUGH. No advertisement, no website, nothing to sell. She wanted people to read it and know that someone cared enough to buy that billboard space and put that message out there, to counter this pervasive scarcity mindset that pressures us to do more, achieve more, earn more, improve, in order to feel worthy.

I told her it was a fantastic idea, but I was concerned that people would not understand it. But I was wrong. A year later, she has *fifteen* billboards up in Los Angeles and Silicon Valley. She hears from people who see one of the billboards, copy down the message, and then find her and share how powerful it was. It seems to especially resonate with people with depression and suicidality—a number of people have reached out to tell her that the message saved them. She's currently working with organizations that want to sponsor more billboards with the affirmation. Cathy herself has struggled with anxiety and depression, and this message—you are enough—has helped her.

"I wanted to give folks a hug," she said. "Now folks are with me doing the same thing, spreading billboards with our

Purpose campaign."[20] She hopes there will be at least one in each state.

When your core sense of self-worth is validated or diversified, you won't be threatened so easily by stress. You can be *challenged* by it . . . and that's exactly what we want.

TODAY'S PRACTICE

DON'T RUN . . . ROAR

Go-Bag Skill: Meet the Moment and Recover Well

Take a moment right now and think of an upcoming event you feel worried about. This could be an important meeting, a presentation, a project. It could also be a small but common daily hassle—being in traffic, going to a social event, or having an argument. Think about why it is stressful to you, what is at stake here. Now, thinking about this event, do the following:

Create a Stress Shield: Your Personal Prescription to Inoculate Yourself against Stress

You can block threat stress from getting into your cells by giving yourself a shield of confidence. So, we will focus on your resources to cope with this particular situation and build those up.

On the next page, jot down three or more reasons you are prepared for this event: you can include skills, resources, or support from other people, or recall similar times you made it through something like this. List the reasons you have what it takes to handle this situation. You are not sure you believe that? Well, believe this: just that thought has the power to make it more likely. Approach the stressful event through a lens of confidence and competence: *I have what it takes to do this.*

Stress Shield: I've Got This Because . . .

_____

_____

_____

_____

_____

_____

_____

_____

_____

_____

_____

_____

After writing down your stress shield statements, close your eyes and imagine yourself in the situation you were stressed about, as vividly as possible. With these stress shield statements in mind, imagine a positive outcome where you've done the very best you can.

Bonus Practices

Remember who you are, from the big-picture perspective: Thinking about this stressful event you have coming up, bring into your mind a few core values you embody, ones that have nothing to do with this situation (see the core values box on page 81). Your multidimensional identity can dampen that feeling of threat from this particular situation.

Get some time perspective—zoom out: Look back on this event (even though it hasn't happened yet!) through the reflective eyes of future you. How much will this affect you in one year? Five years? Ten years? Most of the time the answer is that this event will likely have no impact on our lives in one year. There is always the chance that it will—in which case stakes are truly high, but even so, remind yourself: we can only do our best, and give up control over the rest.

Troubleshooting

When Threat Stress Is Hard to Shake

Using challenge statements, perspective shifts, and values affirmations helps us ruminate less and resolve situations in our minds. These practices can help us feel calm, reduce extra cortisol during the run-up to the event—the common anticipatory stress—so we can be in the moment, be the lion if that's what is required. But sometimes our body doesn't cooperate and we get the full-blown anxiety, panic, racing heart—then what? In the moment, try these tactics from this chapter:

Use your body's energy! That feeling of stress you're experiencing when you are in the thick of it—nervous energy, a surge of adrenaline, the mind whirring, elevated heart rate—can be an asset, energizing and empowering, especially if you frame it that way to yourself. Visualize what your body is doing as it mounts a challenge response: It is sending more blood and oxygen to your heart and to your brain. It's boosting your energy by making extra glucose available. It's building a mindset of positive and creative energy. It's setting up the conditions for you to focus and do what's needed for you to succeed. This is *regenerative energy,* not exhausting burnout energy. Remind yourself: *This stress is a potent energetic resource that's going to help me do well. My body is excited!* Choose that positive thought or another challenge statement from this chapter, or make your own—**you are becoming the lion.**

From "Why me?" to "Try me!" We worked on this in Day 1, but as we discussed, we can never stop having expectations. Hopefully we get better at noticing when we're overly attached to our expectations and releasing them so that we don't experience a threat response when things don't go as expected. But when that *does* happen, flip the script. If you're feeling like a victim of circumstance (*Why me?*) think instead, *Try me!* Think about all the hard situations you have survived already—all that experience and hard-earned wisdom are embodied in you. Your stress mindset shapes your thoughts and experience of reality—including your physiological responses to events. Approach the situation with the mindset of, *What else do you have for me, universe?* and see how different that may feel.

DAY 4

TRAIN FOR RESILIENCE

EVY POUMPOURAS IS A FORMER SECRET SERVICE SPECIAL AGENT, A career in which you literally have to be ready to take a bullet. Uncertainty is a given; resilience is critical. Poumpouras, who is five feet three inches, with a white-blond ponytail and flawless cat-eye eyeliner, is not to be underestimated: she's protected Bill Clinton, who loved to wade into unvetted crowds, shepherded George W. Bush through the crush of a crowd in Egypt, and traveled the world with Barack Obama. On September 11, 2001, she was at the World Trade Center, and ran into the unfolding disaster instead of away, earning a US Secret Service Medal of Valor for her actions. Today, she's a highly sought-after speaker on mental resilience. Her advice for stressful situations? *Accept and adapt.* Don't fight against circumstances you can't control. Accept reality, adapt quickly, and problem-solve from there.

It's good advice, but easier said than done! How do we help ourselves cultivate this kind of mindset so we're ready when the stress of life is upon us? One of Poumpouras's favorite resilience-building practices is perhaps surprisingly simple: she takes cold showers.

Why would this help? Well, Poumpouras has said she started doing it because she was afraid of the cold. She hated it and found herself avoiding it. But she didn't want to be held back from anything by aversion or fear of discomfort. So she started taking cold showers every day to teach her brain and body that she could get through cold just fine. She felt stronger after.

The science suggests that she *is* stronger after. Stepping under the cold water, she exposes her body to a minor, manageable stressor. Her sympathetic nervous system fires up. But then it recovers. And we believe that in the peak-and-recovery process lies a crucial biological piece of stress resilience.

So far, we've been focusing primarily on how you respond to stressors as they emerge, and how to better manage that response. But a huge part of stress resilience is training yourself for it *before* the s*** hits the fan. You work on your stress response when you're *not* in a moment of high stress. To do this, you stress the body out *on purpose*.

I'm not talking about inducing long-term psychological stress. I'm talking about short, concentrated bursts of acute stress, the kind you can easily and naturally recover from—like a brief bout of exercise or plunging into cold water for a swim. It turns out that exposing the body to manageable positive stress does the *opposite* of what long-term toxic stress does: it improves the health and regenerative life span of your cells, instead of slowly wearing them out. We call this *hormetic* stress.

And it's a word we all should know, because it has to do with harnessing stress for good.

The term *hormetic* refers to something that in a larger dose would be harmful, but in a smaller dose is quite beneficial. Compare drinking coffee all day long with enjoying a single shot of espresso. The former is not so great for you and probably leaves you feeling anxious and jittery; the latter comes with mood- and health-boosting benefits. Stress, we believe, is the same way. You don't want to be awash in stress all day long. You *do* want to take short, intense "shots" of it that will prompt your body to initiate recovery processes that are beneficial for your cells and that help them to be more resilient to future stress.

Hormetic Stress: A Cleanup Crew for Your Cells

Here's what happens with hormetic stress (which is also referred to as hormesis and has some friendlier names like "positive stress"): when we have exposure to short-term manageable stressors, the body turns on different responses than with chronic stress. In the nervous system, we want a sharp on-off switch for our stress response. When the sympathetic response turns on, the parasympathetic response shuts down, and vice versa. So you get that sympathetic nervous system spike, but it's followed by a big swell of activity in the parasympathetic nervous system to help shut off the stress response (called *vagal rebound*). It's this counter-regulatory stress response that helps us recover. And not only recover, but *refresh*. Imagine stepping out of that ice-cold shower and then wrapping yourself in a warm towel: stress and recover. It does feel good, and it's good for your cells.

In the cells, hormetic stress processes can create restoration and rejuvenation.[1] We want a sharp acute stress response to turn on the antiaging machinery in there and press the "self-cleaning" button for your cells. Hormesis triggers autophagy, a process in which the cells activate their cleanup crew, gobbling up waste from the day's metabolic processes and recycling it. For example, in worms, heating them up activates heat shock proteins, which trigger autophagy, and then . . . worm longevity! Slightly heated worms actually live longer.[2] But if you give them too much heat for too long, well, that leads to an early funeral. So there's a sweet spot for hormetic stress.

Hormetic stress works almost like a vaccine—you receive a microdose of the "virus" (stress), and then, later, when you face a large, intense similar stressor, you're essentially inoculated against it. Just as your immune system learns how to recognize and combat a virus, your body learns how to metabolize stress when you meet it. When you encounter stress, your body says, *Hey, I've seen this before. I know how to handle this.*

In the field of stress science, we've actually known for quite a while that exposure to short-term stressors makes organisms more resilient to stress later on. It's one of the reasons we believe that people who've experienced *moderate* adversity early in life often have better stress resilience later on. There are a lot of factors that influence this, of course; childhood adversity, when it's chronic, in the form of long-term instability, poverty, and abuse, can have the opposite effect on health. Many brilliant minds are in the process of studying how adverse childhood experiences affect people's health in adulthood, and what sorts of public policies and healthcare interventions can be put into place to screen for and address the lingering effects of toxic stress in childhood. So when I talk about hormetic stress, I'm not talking about these kinds of damaging circumstances. I mean short-term manageable adversity—in small and repeated doses—the kind that can teach the mind and body how to metabolize and recover from stress.

The Good Kind of Stress, and Where to Get It

Your body *loves* acute stress. This process of peak and recovery—of sympathetic nervous system action followed by parasympathetic nervous system action, triggering cell cleanup and repair—is wonderful for us. In fact, we need it. Just as much as your house needs regular cleaning, so do your cells, and acute stress is one process by which that cleanup happens. We need rest and relaxation, yes, but we also need positive stress. We need both. Especially as we age, we tend to have lower vagal tone at rest, which leads to sluggish autonomic stress responses: we get less of the sharp on-off responses in the branches of the nervous system.[3] This makes getting "positive stress" even more important.

When we give ourselves intentional "shots" of acute stress, repeatedly, we're harnessing our natural ability to become stronger. We know this is beneficial—that it's healthy for the body and that it helps us cope with future stress. In animal studies with organisms like mice and worms, we see that exposure to short bouts of hormetic stress is actually life lengthening.

Of course, there are biological differences between worms and humans. So one of our major quests in the field of stress science has been figuring out exactly what tactics produce the hormetic stress response in the human body.

The theory of positive stress has been around for a while in the field of stress science. In fact, the very first paper I ever wrote and published as a scientist, back in 1998, was on positive responses to stress.[4] Early research on hormetic stress was largely based on individual cells or on animals, and researchers often used unnatural stressors like shock, UV exposure, or chemicals—stressors that humans avoid. But one way that researchers could safely induce a positive hormetic stress response in humans was through exercise.

In lab studies, we've learned that there is cross-stressor resilience: Cells exposed to one type of stress (UV shock) are resilient when exposed to a *different* type of stress (heat). They have changed their cellular machinery to cope with whatever comes their way. They mop up free radicals faster. In other words, cells that are exposed to one type of stress are more able to tackle *any* type of stress!

Now let's see if that applies to humans: If you stress yourself with aerobic activity, do you respond better to psychological stress? Do your cells look younger?

Many studies have compared fit people with sedentary people, and they find that the fit group responds to an acute lab stressor with less anxiety and a lower heart rate.[5] That's exciting, but what about people who aren't "fit" to begin with—can they benefit, stress-wise, from physical training? Dr. Tinna Traustadóttir, from Arizona State University, put sedentary people through an eight-week training, and compared them with age-matched controls.[6] At the end of eight weeks, participants were exposed to a physical stressor that created oxidative stress (a tight blood pressure cuff, applied repeatedly, to induce ischemia). The participants who had gone through eight weeks of training responded to the physiological stressor with less oxidative stress. In short? It worked—their bodies became more resilient to stress.

Dr. Eli Puterman of the University of British Columbia is another exercise researcher whom I often collaborate with. He recruited people who were caring full time for a partner with dementia, a high-stress group that did not manage to exercise much.[7] With the support of a trainer calling them, they exercised forty-five minutes three times a week. Six months later, we found that not only did they self-report better stress resilience[8] (less daily stress, rumination, and depression; more mastery and control), but when we drew their blood to examine their cells, we found longer telomeres.[9] The physical training had worked as a kind of protective shield, at the cellular level, against the chronic stress that they lived with.

Getting Your Shots of Stress

For people who have not worked out in years (which typically includes caregivers and people with depression), it's important to start slowly with some kind of movement like yoga or walking, and gradually ramp up to more aerobic, heart-pumping levels. For everyone else, our goal is making stress resilience truly accessible—even to people who are time pressured or economically pressured, or who are juggling many responsibilities in their lives. So we started looking at a low-time-commitment regimen called *high-intensity interval training*, or HIIT.

A session of HIIT asks you to engage in high-energy, heart-pounding activities for short bursts of time, followed by a brief rest. The point is to rapidly get your heart rate up to about 80 percent of its maximum capacity, with enough intervals of rest so that you can keep it up for a short period of time—about ten minutes. Now, interval training is also nothing new—athletes, especially runners, have been practicing it for about a century as part of their training regimen. But more recently, researchers have found that high-intensity interval training may be the best way to get the most bang for your buck in terms of health benefits relative to time invested.

During the pandemic, trapped in the house, I gave in and bought a Peloton bike. I thought I'd run my own little study on myself and see how HIIT training made me feel. I chose a random virtual workout led by a woman I'd never heard of—Robin Arzón—hopped on the bike, and resolved to give it a whirl. Within five minutes of listening to her instructions, my jaw dropped: she was speaking my language of hormetic stress! Her whole model of motivating participants was full of challenge statements like "Develop a relationship with discomfort, and push toward it; it will make you stronger."

The language of stress resilience hit home for me. I became a fan, and started really looking forward to the workouts—hard as they were. She seemed to me to be a brilliantly intuitive psychologist, but I learned she was actually trained as a lawyer and left that career to become a physical trainer. I watched as her worldwide audience grew to reach fifty thousand people at once. Clearly, I wasn't the only one getting hooked on this resilience mindset experience.

We're excited about HIIT as a potential way to improve stress resilience. It is a low-time-commitment, low-cost, fairly straightforward exercise that people can do at home, immediately, to start improving their stress resilience and triggering that health-boosting "cleanup crew" in the body's cells. At the same time, our knowledge of how to induce hormesis has been, for so long, limited to physical exercise, the only vetted strategy that we've run through the rigorous hoops of double-blind studies where we could say, "This clearly creates positive stress and is good for you long-term." I spent two days at the National Institutes of Health with leading stress scientists to discuss how we could best build and measure stress resilience. The only thing everyone agreed upon was . . . exercise. I've walked out of these meetings both pleased that exercise is so highly viewed but shocked that this is still all we know. I go back to my own lab thinking, *That's it? Exercise is all we have?*

The efficacy of HIIT is a solid development—honing exercise down to the "minimum required dose" makes it more accessible. But not everybody can move their bodies in this way. I'd been searching for other ways to create healthy, acute stress in the human body; ways that people could induce a hormetic stress response that *weren't* exercise based. I'd been chewing on the question a long time—basically since I wrote that first resilience paper in 1998!

And that's when I crossed paths with the Iceman.

Lessons from the Iceman

When the Spa Industry Association invited me to the Global Wellness Summit in 2017, I almost said no. It struck me as an insider "wellness industry" event, and I didn't really see how I would fit in or contribute. I was time pressured at the lab and loath to carve out the chunk of days necessary for the travel. On the plane ride to Florida, I started feeling angst and regret about the decision to go. I was going to be a total fish out of water—my work fit in better at conferences on poverty, trauma, and health disparities. Should I be using my time this way? Finally, I cut through the chatter and reminded myself: *There's always something worthwhile that comes out of any conference; I should treat it as an adventure.* I closed my eyes and tried to shift to an open mind about the unknowns ahead, what I might see and learn, and whom I might meet.

I arrived at the conference and prepared for my presentation. The time came for my session, and I was ready to run through it in my head. But the speaker who preceded me grabbed my attention as soon as he walked onstage. He looked a bit like a caveman: tall, wiry, tanned, and wind-whipped, with a big silver beard. He wore shorts and a plain T-shirt. Everyone else in the room was in suits and ties. He was a complete anomaly here. My interest was officially piqued.

His name is Wim Hof, and he's better known by his nickname, "the Iceman." He gained international notoriety for his extreme stunts, most of which involve intense cold exposure: Hiking part of Mount Everest wearing nothing but shorts. Running a marathon, barefoot, in the arctic circle. Sitting in an ice bath for hours. He spent much of his life experimenting with how his body could withstand cold exposure. And, to my delight, his talk was about his own experiences building stress resilience through being in cold or ice for long periods.

He described being "drawn to the ice" since he was a teenager, flinging himself into an icy lake in winter and then feeling strangely invigorated afterward. As an adult, he lost his wife to suicide. He was suddenly a single father of four, struggling financially. And one of the ways he coped, to become more psychologically resilient, was by going deep into nature and by immersing himself in extreme cold: ice-cold water. "My kids saved me," he said. "The ice healed me."

Sounds like a metaphor, but in this case, it may very well be literally true. Hof has been the subject of scientific fascination for years: he has shown it is actually possible for the mind to triumph over the autonomic nervous system in dramatic ways. Researchers have been very interested in Hof's capacity to control processes that we've always thought of as involuntary—like inflammatory responses. It would be easy to write it all off as a fluke—maybe it's just that this one guy has a really incredible nervous system, for whatever reason. But then a couple of studies emerged that took Wim Hof's method (which combines cold exposure and a type of breathing involving deep inhales, powerful exhales, and breath-holding) and looked to see if the benefits he claimed were transferable to others. And . . . they were.

Scientists in the Netherlands (Hof's home country), Drs. Matthijs Kox and Peter Pickkers, injected Hof with an endotoxin (a toxin from bacteria) with the goal of watching his involuntary immune response. He did his breathing practice beforehand, to prepare his body for a resilient stress response. Hof showed significantly less pro-inflammatory response than other people who were injected with the same endotoxin.[10] Then, the researchers trained ten healthy young men to do the ice exposure and breathing techniques over four days. They had the same response Hof did: less inflammatory response after the endotoxin.[11] They had altered the autonomic processes (inflammatory response, immune response, stress response) in their bodies in a very short period of time. This was not about just one person with an unusual nervous system out there hiking Everest in a T-shirt. This was something that could be taught, that potentially anybody could do. It was what I had been seeking for years, and it had just fallen right into my lap. Could Wim Hof's method promote emotional stress resilience and hormesis?

After our presentations were over, Wim Hof and I talked, and he described his training program—how he guides people through breathing and cold-exposure practices. A couple also at the conference, who'd recently started a foundation specifically to investigate exercise and other integrative treatments (non-pharma) for mental health, joined our conversation. They were so intrigued that they offered to fund a study right away, to look at the impact of Hof's method on improving mental health.

I flew home feeling glad that I'd gone to the summit. I'd tolerated uncertainty by choosing curiosity, and I had allowed experience to come to me. It paid off: My collaborators back at UCSF, Wendy Mendes and Aric Prather, were always open to a good rigorous study, especially testing models of positive stress. We ran the study, and we are still assaying blood and scoring data. But in terms of mental health, it appears the Wim Hof method over three weeks may be just as effective as aerobic exercise at reducing stress and depression. It was striking that these processes of briefly stressing the body out—through controlled breathing or through exposure to cold water—had such significant emotional benefits as exercise, the well-studied hormetic stressor safe for humans and known to improve mood. Further, the Wim Hof method appeared superior at instilling positive mood. Those who practiced it felt more positive emotions at the end of each day during the three weeks they practiced, compared to before they started, and compared to those who exercised.

Wim Hof might be the best at sitting in ice baths for hours or climbing Kilimanjaro in shorts. But many people have tried his techniques and report benefits. And there are many ancient practices that involve similar exposures to heat, cold, and breathing (like Tibetan Tummo breathing). The health and resilience benefits of repeated acute stress practices are accessible to anyone. We can all "turn on" hormesis in our bodies. It doesn't take an enormous amount of time or effort, and the payoff can be huge.

Lynne Brick has lived through the transformative benefits of acute stress practices, and has made them daily habits. Years ago, she worked as a trauma nurse. Her work with patients was intense: to qualify for admittance into the shock trauma unit, patients needed to present with multisystem injuries such as head trauma, spinal cord injuries, fractures, or a ruptured spleen. Her job involved trying to save lives and then communicating with upset and grieving families and with doctors and other nurses under extreme pressure. It was a nonstop adrenaline rush—both positive and negative.

Positive: she was working long days helping patients survive and thrive after injury, and it was rewarding.

Negative: the mental stress of making nonstop, high-stakes decisions utilizing the nursing process (assess, diagnose, plan, implement, evaluate); the physical stress of standing eight to twelve hours a day, sometimes with little or no time to take a break or go to the bathroom; and the emotional stress of losing a patient even after all their efforts to save the patient's life. All this stress was exhausting, and it took a toll.

Lynne started coping through exercise—tennis, biking, ballet. The positive effects on her stress levels, her experience of her job, and her experience of life came fast. Suddenly, she says, she understood the medicinal power of movement.

"Movement helped me disassociate from the intensity and trauma of what I experienced each workday," she says now. "Movement helped me to find energy and joy in each day. Movement helped me to be a kinder person to my family and to myself."

Exercise felt so rewarding that Lynne decided to become an aerobics instructor. She learned on the job, teaching herself how to be an effective instructor, then started offering classes to others wanting to become aerobics instructors—locally, nationally, and globally. Along with her partner, Victor, they made fitness their life's business—they eventually became the owners of many Planet Fitness gyms. She has since incorporated heat (infrared sauna) and cold (immersion in the ocean near her home) exposure to her life, along with deep relaxation techniques like slow breathing. Is it sometimes hard to make the time? Sure. But as Lynne says, "I knew if I wanted to keep helping others, I needed to help myself. I needed to put my own oxygen mask on first. I needed to make time for it every day."

Lynne and Victor have had their share of traumatic situations in their lives, including the loss of a family member due to mental illness. Exercise, she says, has influenced every aspect of her life—but especially her response to stress.

Stress Your Body Out On Purpose

Here's what we know. When it comes to triggering hormesis in the body, exercise—any physical activity—works. It's the long-standing classic. But we now know that very *brief* bouts of physical activity—like high-intensity interval training—will also trigger this beneficial recovery process.

It's not about precisely what you do or how long you do it. You don't need to exercise for an hour. You only need to stress the body out *just enough* so that it "turns on" the recovery process.

You want the parasympathetic swell, the vagus nerve activation, the internal cell cleanup. And as it turns out, Wim Hof has really been onto something all this time when it comes to the power of hormetic stress to trigger the natural rejuvenating ability of our cells: you can also get this effect by exposing yourself to cold for just a few minutes, or practicing certain types of hypoxic breathing with expert guidance (don't overdo it!).

Here's how hypoxic breathing works: it's basically a type of cyclical hyperventilation. You take deep, vigorous, fast inhales, followed by powerful exhales . . . but not all the way. You inhale quickly, slowly exhale; then repeat. On Hof's YouTube channel, he offers guidance on this breathing method. People sometimes experience mild sensations with hypoxic breathing; others report feeling light-headed, warm, or even euphoric. After about thirty to fifty vigorous breaths, you take a big inhale, exhale partway, and then hold your breath as long as you can without feeling dizzy or faint. You might start with thirty seconds, although people get better at this and can eventually go for as long as two minutes. You do about three cycles of this—the hypoxic breathing and then the breath holding. And that's it. What you're doing is shifting from low to high blood oxygen, and causing many other changes in the blood: an ideal cocktail of hormetic stress.

Drs. Kox and Pickkers first drew blood while people were doing hypoxic breathing in the lab, and the tests show a natural spike in epinephrine—that's part of the stress response to hypoxia. Your body's saying, *I can't breathe, mobilize a big stress response!* The higher the epinephrine spike, the better the anti-inflammatory response later. In other words: the intensity of the beneficial "refresh and repair" response is yoked to the intensity of the stress. A cold shower works essentially in the same way: you shock your system, throw it into acute stress, and then reap the benefits as your body "recovers" from the stressor. Since that first study by Drs. Kox and Pickkers, one small study found that for people with an inflammatory type of arthritis, the method appeared to reduce levels of inflammation in the blood.[12]

When I tried Hof's breathing method, I felt immediately different afterward. I felt like a placid lake—you could not agitate me. I was feeling ease with a buzz of energy. As the day went on, I felt more impervious to stressors that normally might have thrown me for a bit of a loop. When we use hormetic stress methods, we can shrink our stress, make it more malleable, change how we see it so we feel more excited than threatened by it. For me, it is often the *body-up* methods, more than the *top-down* methods, that are stronger, that cut through my mind chatter and any tension I am holding in my muscles. In other words, we often try to rely on the mind to think our way out of our stress—but the body is built to help us metabolize stress; we should use it too. If you feel like you have layers of stress stored in your body that you need to get at, exposing yourself to some brief "shots" of stress may allow you to metabolize the stored stress out of your body. You ice it, you heat it, you breathe it out. You change its physical properties so it moves through your body in a productive, healthy, refreshing way.

The bottom line: you can put your body through *any* of these positive stress experiences (if done safely) and build resilience. That said, many of these positive stress practices are not well studied except for exercise; I am generalizing here about hormetic stressors, so you will have to experiment wisely. We know for sure that in worms many types of stressors repeated at moderate doses promote cell-healthy hormesis and longevity; in humans, short, repeated bodily stress may very well promote stress resilience, but this is a new field, and there is still much to discover about what types of stressors are healthy, which doses are optimal, and which are harmful. HIIT in particular is extremely effective at not only making people *feel* better but also really improving the nervous system response and the immune system, and promoting growth factors in both the brain and body that help with restoration from stress.

We don't want to be experiencing low-level stress all the time—the human body wasn't built for that constant yellow mind state. It was built to experience acute red mind stress and then recover afterward with some green mind relaxation. And we can't get to recovery unless we intentionally put our bodies through a positive stress experience—even just a short one will do the trick.

So today, that's exactly what we're going to do.

TODAY'S PRACTICE

A SHOT OF HEALTHY STRESS

Go-Bag Skill: Use Your Stress Response for Health and Longevity

When we train the body to metabolize stress well by giving it "doses" of positive hormetic stress, we become more instinctually resilient to stressors as they come along. Today we teach the body to respond to stress with an acute peak response, and then recover quickly with restorative parasympathetic action and cell cleanup. If you are up for this, I suggest trying it in the morning, when your diurnal rhythm calls out for activity (high cortisol, high glucose).

"Stress fitness" means exercising the body with short bursts of stress several times a week. We have several options for this type of positive physical stress, any of which will produce a healthy hormetic response in the body. The best way is to push ourselves to a little bit of discomfort with either brief, intense exercise or cold exposure. The Wim Hof breathing method is also very effective, but it takes a bit of practice and can cause light-headedness. You are welcome to try it—guidance is easily accessible on his YouTube channel. Note that it may be a good choice for people who cannot exercise (due to disability or other reasons). But for today, if you can, consider choosing from one of these two methods.

Choose your challenge . . .

Option 1: HIIT It!

Try one round of high-intensity interval training. Don't worry—it sounds tougher than it is! One cycle of HIIT takes roughly seven minutes. The basic rules: Choose a selection from the following list of exercises. You can pick as many as you like, but keep it simple to start.

An important note: If you haven't been active in a while, don't start with HIIT! Skip the chart below and start with something accessible like slow to brisk walking. The idea is the same: move toward the top of your capacity and stay there for a few minutes. Add music to keep it brisk, use a step tracker, or include a partner—whatever will make it joyful for you! You can experience the stress benefits of physical movement in many ways.

If you do try HIIT: I recommend searching online for a seven-minute guided HIIT video (plenty of options should pop up). If you do this on your own, simply choose three exercises and then rotate between them. Set your phone time for seven minutes. Start your favorite upbeat music if it helps you stay motivated, and begin. Do each exercise for thirty seconds, followed by ten seconds of rest. Repeat, with different or the same exercises, until the seven minutes are up.

Jumping Jacks	Wall Sit	Push-Ups	Knee Push-Ups
Plank	Knee Plank	Crunches	Step-Ups
Squats	Triceps Push-Ups	Knees Up	Lunges

If you're not familiar with some of these exercises, you can find videos online as well as many guided versions of the preceding workout (type "7-minute workout" into your internet search engine).

The workout is highly customizable—this is your seven minutes to stress your body out in a healthy, positive way. You do not have to be "good" at exercise, or at any particular level of physical fitness, to benefit from this. At the same time, you could be a top athlete and *not* benefit if you don't push yourself a little.

No matter which exercises you choose or what your physical capacity or experience, your mission is the same: Find your edge, where you feel some discomfort or struggle. Welcome the discomfort and difficulty as part of the experience—don't fight against it. Focus on *this* thirty seconds—then you get to rest. Then focus on the next thirty seconds. Focus on what your body is doing in this specific moment: burning through stress metabolically with this effort. Your body loves this!

Option 2: Turn the Dial to Cold

You don't have to run barefoot through the arctic to reap the hormetic benefits of a cold shock to the system. Today, at the end of your usual warm shower, turn the dial to cold—as cold as you can stand it. Can you stay under the cold stream for fifteen or thirty seconds? A minute? We had our research participants stay in the cold water for up to three minutes. Push yourself to your edge, in exactly the same way you would with exercise, and then: *relax into it.*

This is key. You'll feel the urge to tighten up, clench, re-sist, cringe, and gasp for air—being immersed in cold water is uncomfortable! It's shocking! That's *exactly* how we re-spond to sudden unexpected stressors in a way that leaves us struggling to get through them and recover. With phys-ical stress, we can realize that we *don't* need to have a psy-chological stress response, too, and that helps us recover from the stress sooner. In a cold shower, you can grit your teeth and tense your shoulders and just bear it . . . or, you can use this precious moment to build stress resilience. Match the shock of the stress response with a relaxed mind as much as possible. This is what builds resilience.

You can end your warm shower with cold water (and you will find your body warms up from the inside) or, if you pre-fer, start with cold and end with hot. This is best done in the morning so you can enjoy the shot of energy for the day— but each person responds differently.

Remind yourself: *My body loves this. My body needs this. My body was built for this.*

With both option 1 and option 2, what we're shooting for is a feeling of being energized. Of being able to "seize the day." You are actively training yourself to "be the lion," as we discussed in the previous chapter. The more you *train* for resilience before stress occurs, the more prepared you'll be to meet it and process it in a healthy, effective way. As one woman in our Wim Hof study reported, "I have more coping energy. I can just deal with things so much better."

Along with bodily stress resilience comes emotional resilience—they go hand in hand. Tolerating cold and discomfort and pushing ourselves to the edge of our physical comfort zone gets us used to tolerating unpleasant emotions as well. It doesn't mean that we don't feel unpleasant emotions—it means we handle and metabolize them better when we do have them.

Both of these options are like meditation, in a way: we focus our attention on the body, on finding our edge of discomfort, and on feeling *in control* of this beneficial acute stress response.

Bonus Practice

Heat It Up!

Cold exposure turns on positive hormetic stress . . . and so does heat exposure, in the right circumstances. This is in the "extra-credit" section because the best way to try positive stress heat exposure is to use a sauna. And not everyone is going to have easy immediate access to one of those! However, if you do and are interested in trying this, it *is* an option along with the other strategies we've already gone over.

We have a wealth of research showing the emotional and physical benefits of sauna use. "Hyperthermia" is effective for turning on hormetic stress in the body. For example, within around thirty minutes of sauna use, heat shock proteins increase, and if you do this repeatedly, they remain higher than in non-heat-acclimated people. Your heart rate increases during the sauna, as if you were doing moderate exercise. In humans, regular sauna use reduces blood pressure and improves cardiovascular function indices, similar to the effects of exercise.[13] We know some of the mechanisms: In mice with heart disease (being fed a diet equivalent to McDonald's food), repeated heat treatments turned on heat shock proteins, which activated anti-inflammatory pathways and led to improvements in their atherosclerosis, and even a longer life.[14]

Hyperthermia may also help treat depression.[15] Researchers first found that a single sauna session of an hour to an hour and half, which can typically bring people's core temperature up to about 103 degrees, improved symptoms of depression for up to six weeks after.[16] This was exciting, because effective treatments for depression are hard to come by.

People with depression often also have dysregulation in their thermoregulation systems. By putting them in a hyperthermia situation in which we *force* the body to turn on these cooling mechanisms (the body's natural response to being artificially heated up is to try to cool itself down), we also "turn on" this mechanism that hasn't been working properly. The more the reduction in core body temperature in the days after heating, the more relief people had from their depression. In her research[17] on hyperthermia mechanisms so far, Dr. Ashley Mason, an associate professor here at UCSF, has found that an easily accessible standard commercial infrared sauna that one can order online (as opposed to an expensive medical-grade infrared sauna) can reduce depressive symptoms. Although we need more research, sauna use is looking like a unique way you can trigger hormetic stress in your body and improve your mood and health.

Troubleshooting

If HIIT Doesn't "Hit" Right Away . . .

If you tried option 1 today, you might not feel a lot of positive effect the very first time you do it. In fact, expect the first week to be the hardest. However, if you do this regularly (just seven to fourteen minutes several times a week), you *will* build up stress resilience in the cardiovascular and nervous systems, and you'll build up more positive emotions in response to the exercise. Your body will quickly begin to learn: *This feels good. I feel better after exercise.* As with any new habit, give your body a chance to get used to this one so you can really feel the benefits in your day-to-day.

If You're Struggling with Depression . . .

Any kind of exercise, even short commitments like HIIT, is really effective for treating depression. The problem is, when you're depressed, you just don't feel like exercising. It can feel impossible to work up the motivation. If you're someone who experiences more serious states of depression or anxiety, and you feel held back from trying out these methods, here's what we know: There's a barrier at the beginning. It doesn't feel good. But you may be able to get beyond the initial obstacle of feeling "blah." Know that any movement, even for five minutes to start, is meaningful and significant to your brain. Gentle yoga may be a great choice. If you can, try hiring a personal coach. Or ask a friend or neighbor to be a motivational partner—do it together for a week. Text each other, check in, give each other prompts and encouragement. It goes a long way to be accountable to someone else, and to feel like you have a partner in this process.

If You Have High Anxiety . . .

From a mental health perspective, there is some nuance as to which types of mental health conditions exercise can help. A practice like HIIT is great for depression, but it may be challenging for someone on the higher end of the anxiety spectrum. For some, exercise and other hormetic stressors may make them more anxious.

If you tend to experience anxiety strongly in your body, and you know this about yourself, you might find that the HIIT exercise makes your anxiety worse rather than better. That said, I still recommend that you try a hormetic stress practice at a slow pace, because it may be that after a few attempts, as it becomes more familiar and less of an "unknown threat," your body will gradually adjust, getting used to the physiological changes that can feel like anxiety (like the racing heartbeat). This can eventually help reduce your anxiety. But if it's not the right choice for your particular mind and body state, respect that reality and be kind to yourself about it. A different method, like cold showers or a sauna, might be a better fit for your body.

DAY 5

LET NATURE
DO THE WORK

IMAGINE THIS: FOR OVER A YEAR, YOU ARE COMMANDED TO STAY HOME.
Everything closes; there is no place to go. You do all your work
via computer, bathed in the blue light of your laptop or monitor.
There is no socializing. You can communicate or interact with
others only through the big screen of your computer or the
small screen of your phone.

Too familiar, I know. Unless you were a first responder or
essential worker (which came with its own unique and intense
stressors), this was probably your reality for at least part of the
pandemic. We were inside a lot, staring at our screens for the
majority of the day: suddenly, it was where we did everything
from working to socializing to collaborating with colleagues.
There was no other way. Even before the pandemic, the amount
of time that we were all spending inside, away from the light of
day and the rhythms of the earth we live on, was already at a
historic high. Now, the more we were in front of screens for
work, the more frequently we were checking news, social

media, and other sources of global bad news. Across the board, surveys revealed unprecedented levels of anxiety, depression, sleep problems, and burnout.

During lockdowns, there was a common way that people coped with pandemic anxiety: they went outside, into nature. With everything closed, it became the only option for getting out of our houses and taking a break. Studies have since measured how much "blue-green space" people were getting—exposure to urban parks, woods, rivers, and coastal areas. A survey conducted by the UK's Mental Health Foundation showed that 62 percent of people in the UK reported finding relief by going for a walk in urban gardens and parks.[1] And there appeared to be a dose-response effect: the more time outdoors in the natural world people got, of any age (the survey looked at people of all ages, from children to older adults), the better their mental health. In Spain, during the initial COVID-19 wave when the country was under a strict lockdown, those without views of or access to nature had much worse mental health, regardless of income.[2] Nature, it seemed, was a powerful antianxiety drug.

I live in a city, and I have a city mind—I am habituated to the ambulances, fire engines, and car motor sounds, all of which surely add to my yellow mind state of vigilance, even though I'm no longer aware of it. Every day, I take my dog for a walk. No matter how busy I am, there's no option to skip it. I have to set aside my to-do list and just go. I walk him out by the ocean, where I can hear the waves, or in Golden Gate Park among the trees, where the musical rustle of wind in the leaves causes me to—however briefly—forget my worries and snap into attunement with the world around me. The contrast reminds me, I need more nature! And the effects of *raw* nature—when I can get away from the city completely and immerse myself in a wild place—are even more powerful.

My favorite escape is to a remote house by the ocean. Within a day my nervous system recalibrates, just by being close to the wild, open ocean. My thoughts move away from the ruminative loops about work and family and toward the rhythmic, transfixing sound of the waves. All my problems seem to shrink in comparison with the stunning enormity of the Pacific. My body seems to synchronize with the environment around me. Whereas at home I am in sync with the digital clock and the screens that run my life and work, here I am attuned to the sunrise, the sunset, the changing temperature of the day, the scents, sounds, and sensations.

If there was a silver lining of the pandemic, maybe it was this: during one of the most stressful and uncertain times that any of us have experienced in our lives, people were forced outside into nature, when it was accessible. Sure, it was by necessity—we really had no other options!—but it turns out that exposure to nature, in all forms and contexts, is one of the most powerful and immediate ways to shrink stress.

Here's the problem: Most of us are now back in "nature deficit." In our regular day-to-day, in our typical routines, we experience overstimulation and loss of perspective. We quite literally get lost inside the minutiae of our problems. In an effort to solve them, we focus on them more, and they get bigger and bigger. The stress becomes enormous, filling the whole lens. It's all we can see.

When Stress Creates Cognitive Overload: Yellow Mind

The human brain works as a master prediction machine: based on our past experiences, our memories, and our body's signals, we are constantly predicting what the next moments will bring. So if we're frequently overconnected to screens and electronics, the result is that we're always anticipating massive amounts of stimuli to be forthcoming. We expect it. We get hooked to it. We even seek it.

With this habit and expectation of being connected, engaged, and stimulated, it can feel impossible for us to shift into a more peaceful state, doing less, or nothing. The brain tells us we should be doing something, worrying about this or that, checking the news or email, and on and on and on. In red or yellow mind, our minds prefer to do *anything* other than sit in stillness. In one study,[3] people were left to think freely for ten minutes or more. If the participants wanted something to do during that period, they could choose to administer a minor electric shock to themselves. Almost 20 percent of the participants self-administered a minor shock: some were curious, but some did it out of a drive to escape boredom or their own thoughts.

Because of this overconnection to stimuli, and a cultural drive to overwork, we tend to be inside most of the day, and in front of screens. When we lose in-person connection to others while we have big doses of social media, it's a deadly formula. Social networks thrive on negative emotions and angry emojis; that's what gets amplified.[4] And now we know that Facebook algorithms have been making that problem even worse, spreading material with angry emojis five times more than those with Likes.[5] Then there's the way that social media is set up to make us believe everyone else is living a more ideal life than we are, an effect that hits our youth the hardest: suicide rates in US teens stayed stable from 2000 to 2007 and then increased 57 percent by 2018.[6] Technology addiction is reflected in some of the policies trying to rein it in—France, for example, has passed a "right to disconnect from email" law so that people can unplug at night and not have to answer urgent work emails—but most of us don't have this protection. Rather, we suffer from the aforementioned disconnection syndrome—we're disconnected from ourselves, from how we feel, from our bodies, from each other, and from nature.

Urbanites may suffer from this even more. Those of us who live in urban environments get used to a certain constant level of stimulation, but that doesn't mean it's not affecting us. "The urbanicity effect" refers to the higher rates of depression, anxiety, and schizophrenia in people who grow up in urban areas, who also tend to overreact to social stressors compared with people who grow up in rural areas.[7] Even urban honeybees are different from rural honeybees—they have greater levels of oxidative stress, presumably from the higher levels of pollution, noise, and other stimulants.[8]

We live in a world where there is simply too much going on—too much stimuli from our screens, too much constant engagement, too many distracting pulls on our attention. But our mental state and stress levels are shaped by our environment. By going into nature, we use this to our advantage.

Let Nature Calibrate Your Nervous System

It's simple: By shifting our physical environment, we can shift our mental state. We can change both the content of our thoughts and our thought processes. For many people, this shift is almost automatic when they place themselves into the natural world: the mind moves from conditioned thought patterns—rapid thoughts, negative self-talk, anticipating what's next—to discursive thought, which is slower, calmer, creative, curious. Immersion in nature immediately reduces the amount of human-created sensory stimuli we are used to—from screens, information, urban sounds. It enforces a mental break. It's a sanctuary environment that calms the mind and eases the body. Yes, we can train the brain to do this in our typical environment (through mindfulness practice, for example, as we discussed), but nature is a quick way to do it, and it comes with a whole host of other benefits for our mental state and nervous system.

The beneficial effects of forests have been well documented. Many studies have shown that regular immersion in forests improves a wide range of health problems. In some countries, it's called *forest bathing*. Forest bathing is an established practice in Asia in particular—researchers in Korea and elsewhere have studied the effect of being immersed in the forest ecosystem for several hours, several times a week, while walking slowly and paying mindful attention to the environment, or sitting and viewing the landscape. In clinical trials it has been shown to reduce blood pressure, cortisol, and inflammation.[9] In New Zealand, doctors will write a "green prescription": *You are recommended to spend two hours in nature, three times a week.* It's so effective, it's been folded into mainstream medicine in many places.

One of the ways forest bathing has this incredible effect on the human nervous system is through our sensory channels: plant or tree odors like cedarwood may reduce biological stress, and in forests, the air is not only less polluted, but more ionized,[10] especially when there are waterfalls or recent rain. Sound plays a big role too: wind in the trees, birdsong, and the sounds of water or ocean are all intrinsically calming and relaxing to humans. We aren't sure exactly why, but one theory is that it taps into old evolutionary feelings of safety. Visually, the same effect may be happening when we are surrounded by shades of green—we may be evolutionarily conditioned to feel calm and safe in this environment. On the flip side of that coin, a more urban landscape can be overstimulating to humans, because instead of natural shapes and horizons, we see and hear too many unnatural shapes and sounds. The urban landscape, for many, doesn't trigger safety—it triggers vigilance and alertness.

This dramatic shift we experience in nature is called the *attentional restoration effect*: we have relieved attentional overload, we have opened up space in our mind, we feel better. Studies have examined brain waves, or brain activity, while people looked at pictures of either nature or urban landscapes. They find that when compared with nature scenes, urban landscapes immediately demand more attention and cognitive processing, and activate stress-related areas like the amygdala.[11] Dr. Pooja Sahni, a researcher at the Indian Institute of Technology in New Delhi, found that when watching a nature video, our brains show greater alpha and theta waves (neural states that create relaxation) and enhanced cognitive ability to overcome distractions.[12] Interestingly, waterfalls and rivers seem to be the most potent nature stimuli in Sahni's study.

The Magic of Water

Many people also resonate with the soothing sound of rhythmic ocean waves—it affects our breathing, slowing it down and encouraging deeper breaths than the shallow and insufficiently oxygenated breathing that is our habit (more on this in the next chapter). And there is something special about water: marine biologist Dr. Wallace Nichols calls this "the Blue Mind effect," and it's exactly what we've been on a mission to achieve this week. "Blue mind," as we've been discussing it in this book, refers to a deeply restful state that generates well-being and restoration, but Nichols's point (in his book also titled *Blue Mind*) is that water is a particularly effective way to achieve well-being. He describes water as medicine. Through water, we may be able to reach blue mind states that we otherwise would not.

Exposure to water—whether it's being in the ocean or a pool, or floating in a saltwater tank—induces psychological benefits of peace and well-being. People have used water for centuries for health: from hot to cold, from natural hot springs to highly engineered indoor float tanks. Float tanks are filled with water and large quantities of salt so that your body can safely and effortlessly float. People report that in these tanks, they feel a pervasive sense that all their needs are met, that they are safe and at ease. One group has been studying the effects of tank flotation with *silence*, a powerful way to change your mental context by stripping away auditory stimuli, and found that with a single ninety-minute float tank session, people with high anxiety or anxiety disorders saw their anxiety levels come down close to that of the average person.[13]

Why? One theory is that floating in water may change the body's signals, dramatically reducing muscle tension and blood pressure, which then has ripple effects throughout the body and mind. Floating in water also seems to increase *interoception*, the connection between our sensory awareness and our body. Attention turns inward—not toward ruminative thought processes, but toward the breath, the heartbeat, the feelings and sensations in the body. Blood pressure goes down by, on average, ten points, and the more it lowers, the more serenity people feel—a calm that lasts all day.

We walk around with an enormous cognitive load. We're

carrying so much around in our working memory—worries and to-dos, thoughts that pop up out of nowhere, reactions to the stimuli around us. In nature, our attention is more effortlessly focused. Our attentional control improves. In the lab, we see this happen on neuropsychological tests. The cognitive load is relieved, opening up space for creativity, spontaneous thought, and present-moment experience. This all loops back to what we've been talking about throughout this book: that we are unconsciously stressed most of the time. We're taxed in ways we aren't even aware of. People often don't realize how stressed they are until they get into nature and notice the *absence* of stress for the first time in a long time. A close friend of mine who absolutely loves her life in San Francisco said recently after a weekend away in the woods, "I didn't even know it, but the city is so stressful!"

Getting to Blue Mind

As humans, we have an affinity for nature—being in nature allows us to access green mind states of relaxation and even blue mind states. Blue mind can be a state of deep relaxation (as we discussed in the introduction), but it can also show up as a moment of transcendence in which you feel connected to your body and environment and experience a calm expansiveness of thought. In fact, immersive nature exposure is one of the quickest ways to achieve a blue mind state.

I've been studying stress resilience for decades now, and quite honestly I am amazed by how effective immersion in nature is at shaping the activity of the autonomic nervous system. Nature is unique in its capacity to soothe, to calm, to put things into perspective, and to shrink stressors that once seemed huge. A major part of this is because we experience feelings of wonder and awe from the raw beauty of the natural world.

Exposure to nature puts us into contact with beauty and with a world that is so much larger than us. When polled, people who seek out nature describe being powerfully impacted by the "vastness" of the ocean, the "massive" size of the mountains, the "enormity" of the desert landscape or the open sky. What seems to bring people calm, peace, and relief from stress is a shift in perspective that comes from the sheer scale of the natural world; being in nature reminds us of our relatively small size in the larger context of the universe.

Dacher Keltner, a professor of psychology at the University of California, Berkeley, is an emotions researcher whom I have known for twenty years. Early in his career he focused very narrowly on one positive emotion: awe.

I didn't understand his fascination back then, but now it seems like one of the most important human experiences to understand. He has continued to do extensive research into what he calls the "uniquely human experience of awe" and has found that when we feel awe, we experience immediate biological effects, like better heart rate variability, reduced blood pressure, and a measurable drop in stress levels. In older adults, a simple "awe walk" (noticing things, taking photos together) versus a typical walk led to lower daily stress and greater daily positive emotions and, in their photos, larger smiles.[14] Awe is transformative—the feeling of being in the presence of something larger than oneself immediately snaps things into perspective for us. When we are reminded of the grandeur of the world, issues that seemed large and looming, driving up stress in the body, suddenly shrink. Our worries simply cannot compete.

Keltner believes that awe may turn out to be a powerful "prescription" for things like stress, anxiety, depression, and PTSD. His center ran a study in which they took veterans with PTSD into the wilderness. Over the course of a single week, they saw a *30 percent* drop in PTSD symptoms.

"People have been writing about awe since the beginning of human time," says Keltner. "Awe is when we encounter vast things we don't understand. Lab studies show that our sense of self gets smaller. We feel we are connected to larger things, like ecosystems. We get really curious about the world. Our minds open. Awe makes us committed to the community we share; we put aside our differences and become more interested in other people. The data are coming in, and I actually think that awe is potentially the most central pathway to healing and resilience that we can find."

Awe: A Long-Lasting Anti-stress Medicine?

Keltner's research into awe and human resilience is ongoing, and one of the questions he's investigating is how long the effects of awe last. We know that awe experiences not only reduce stress, but have a neural signature as well—awe can deactivate the brain network that fuels rumination and negative self-related mind wandering. But is it lasting? Is it fleeting and transient, working only in that moment, or does it have residual effects that stay with you?

My belief is this: it could last a lifetime.

My colleague George Bonanno, a world expert in trauma and author of *The End of Trauma*, had a tough childhood. Growing up, he had to deal with an abusive parent. He moved out as a teenager, got into heavy drugs, and watched his life start to fall apart. At seventeen, he decided to leave his hometown, to get away from patterns of addiction and bad influences and try to start fresh. He started hitchhiking to the West Coast. A friendly truck driver picked George up, learned his story, and ended up driving hundreds of miles out of his way to get George toward his destination. George doesn't remember the man's name, but he remembers what he said: "Kid, what you're doing is absolutely the best thing. You will take control of your life. You will make mistakes. But that's okay, because they'll be *your* mistakes, and you'll learn from them and grow."

By nightfall, the driver had to finally turn around and go back the other direction. He suggested that George walk a little way off the highway and sleep up in the hills—he pointed the way—and then resume hitchhiking in the morning. So George walked up the hill in the pitch black, shook out his sleeping bag, and fell asleep under the stars. When he awoke at dawn, he realized he was right in the middle of a mountain range. He had never seen mountains before in his life. The sky was huge, filled with brilliant pinks and purples, and he had the most overwhelming feeling that he struggles still to describe—he refers to it now as "a sense of God, in some nonconceptual form."

"At that moment I saw a clear order to the universe," he says now, so many decades later. "Timeless, not good or bad, and felt in touch with it. I knew right then and there that everything was going to be okay. My life would be okay. And literally, from that moment on, my life was okay."

George is now a pioneer in human resilience, and his work has shown that most people, after going through a traumatic event, will bounce back to their previous state of well-being relatively quickly, within a few months, and the vast majority within a year or two. We are resilient. Our bodies, our cells, our spirits are built for resilience. And awe is an ace we have in our pocket—it can cut through hard moments and strengthen inner resilience. You may have had moments when all of a sudden, your life had more purpose; you saw your place in it and how the puzzle pieces all fit together. These insights come when we are in green or blue mind states, rarely red or yellow.

"Experience awe" isn't usually something that shows up on our daily, weekly, or monthly to-do lists. But it needs to be. Keltner told me about a recent period when he forgot about the importance of regular awe-inspiring experiences.[15] In 2019, he lost his younger brother, whom he was extremely close to. Then COVID hit, and with it, the stressors that we all experienced: being cut off from friends and family, worries about illness, uncertainty about the future. Two years went by during which he felt that he was just pushing through with his head down and his teeth gritted. And one day he realized: he felt terrible.

"I felt the constant tension of chronic stress," he says. "I felt the heat of inflammation. My mind was fixated on problems. My cells were probably aging prematurely! And I just had this epiphany: I study awe. I have to go and live it."

It was COVID, so big travel was out of the question. And he had committed to living a low-carbon-footprint life: no big road trips, no flights, no buying lots of stuff. He had to experience awe simply. He started looking for the feeling everywhere. He'd go for a walk and find some new trees he hadn't noticed before. He'd listen to music. He'd watch the sky at sunset. He started reading for pleasure again, to get back to the big ideas that used to broaden his mind and thrill him. And it worked. The grief and worries were still there—they don't go away—but they didn't consume him anymore.

Recalibrate Your Nervous System, No Matter Where You Live

Being connected to nature is not easy for everyone. We tend to like what we grew up with and are acclimated to. For many, being suddenly immersed in raw nature may not be immediately calming, because it's unfamiliar. Those of us who've grown up in a more urban landscape, who have acclimated to its rhythms, sights, and sounds, may initially feel more safe and calm in that familiar busy environment. But I want to suggest that if we give it the chance, if we put some time into acclimating to these green or blue landscapes, there is a deeper part of us that can feel an even more pervasive sense of calm, of focused attention, of a quieted mind, when we are surrounded by the natural world instead of the human-made one. "Full immersion" in nature can provide a kind of "mega-effect," and so I encourage you to give it a try. But when we're talking about managing our day-to-day stress, urban nature also packs a huge punch.

In studies, the presence of urban greenery is associated with better attention, lower heart rate, lower anxiety, and more peacefulness. Meanwhile, low urban greenery is associated with higher violence, worse mental health, lower physical activity, and higher mortality.[16] Children are affected too—higher hyperactivity and behavioral problems are associated with low-nature areas—and this is all controlling for socioeconomic factors.[17] Telomeres seem to like green spaces too! A study out of Hong Kong found that people who lived in the outer suburbs, with more greenery and nature spaces, had longer telomeres than those who lived deeper in the city (again, controlled for socioeconomic factors).[18] Fish from rural rivers have longer telomeres than fish from urban, more polluted rivers.[19] Same thing for rural versus urban birds.[20] There are so many ways that gardens and trees promote well-being and calmness, including in urban spaces.

In a recent conversation with a friend, I belittled urban nature, saying, "I'm starved of nature!" I was comparing my city walks with a long wilderness immersion. My friend gently (and rightly) pointed out to me that nature is everywhere, if I look for it. We build cities on top of nature, and it bursts out joyfully everywhere it can. Birds build their nests in the trees, or wherever they can (gutters, city fire escapes, even in potted plants). Resilient plants spring up from cracks in the asphalt. Gardens explode in tiny patches of lawn or window boxes and other containers. Nature will always seep in, and that's something we can notice and even nurture. I find myself appreciating my garden more than I ever have and opening my sensory channels to all the nature that thrives in the city. I can get daily hits of urban nature that help immensely, while also knowing that I crave and benefit from wild nature. So now I'm going into my backyard every day to feel the ground under my bare feet, to feel the sun on my face, and to hear the birds.

Your Mission Today

Experience nature. Experience awe. Remind yourself of your place in the world. Remind yourself of the real "size" of your problems from a larger perspective. Sensory input from nature sends signals of safety, calmness, and grounding—this is deep and evolutionary. Even urban nature can do this. This is the green mind state.

We were really good at this during the pandemic, and we saw measurable benefits. Let's learn from it. The pandemic was a watershed time in terms of stress science: we learned so much about what really builds stress resilience and leads to greater well-being, greater joy. And nature was a really big piece of it. As people began getting vaccinated, workplaces began to open up again, and life started to shift back—at least for the moment—toward pre-pandemic rhythms, I remember something that my colleague Elizabeth Blackburn, my partner in telomere research, said to me: "Let's not let the pandemic go to waste."

Crisis creates opportunities for change. We call this *posttraumatic growth*. Nature was a coping mechanism commonly used during the pandemic, and we learned from large-scale studies how truly beneficial it is. Let's learn from this. Don't go back inside. Go outside at every opportunity and experience the sensory bath of the natural world, which does wonders for your stress baseline, moving it toward green mind.

There's a stability and a slowness to nature—it's patient and resilient itself, and it inspires that in our bodies as well. Inside, we have the time pressures of our self-constructed day. Outside, we realize that the time frame that matters is measured in years and centuries. You walk in the woods and see that a large tree has fallen and died, and then you notice the new growth, and all the new shoots, the offspring that will grow for the next century. You see the history of the earth, and the future. And I must note here that due to the climate crisis, I also feel sadness and sometimes despair for the threat to nature, and I am sure you do too. We need nature for our well-being, and for our survival, and we need dramatic actions to protect it that we feel will have impact—we'll talk more about this a bit later.

Today we tap into the deep calming power of nature in whatever way is accessible to you. If you can immerse yourself in raw nature today, wonderful. But remember: nature is potent and helpful to you in any form. It's through the sensory channels that nature affects us, so there are many routes we can take. A walk in your neighborhood can work. Going into your backyard can work. You can bring the sounds and smells of nature into your home or office. Whichever method you choose, your mission is to recalibrate the nervous system by using the cues of the natural world. By creating a nature-evoking sanctuary inside, or going outside, you change your context and in doing so, change the processes of your mind and body to be calmer, more joyful, and more resilient. Today, let nature do the work for you.

TODAY'S PRACTICE

LET NATURE SHRINK STRESS

Go-Bag Skill: Get Perspective and Get Connected

Today you can choose from three different options for your practice, depending on your capacity. Whatever you cannot do today, know that you can always try it in the future. Any of these practices will work to shrink stress, recalibrate the nervous system, and give you a calming "reset" to continue on in your day with more resilience.

Option 1: Immersion

Think of someplace you can go today that's raw nature, a place that feels like true wilderness, away from the sights and sounds of human urban life. Today you want to walk in nature for full immersion, attuning your mind outward, noticing both the small details and the visual sweeps. My friend Mark Coleman, who leads regular nature retreats[21] and who is British, likes to call this type of walking "bimbling" about. This is wandering without a goal. You are not trying to get somewhere. You aren't trying to finish a hiking loop or achieve a peak. It is strolling slowly, noticing things as you go.

Ideally go alone. If you're more comfortable with others, that works too. But remember that this is not time to talk and catch up. It's a sensory experience. Walk in silence, slowly, and far apart. Your primary mission is to let your senses be fully engaged. This is a time to become outwardly focused and open to what you see, hear, smell, taste, and feel. Otherwise, it's easy to become immersed in something else: your own spinning thoughts. If you're walking silently, slowly, but your mind is elsewhere, at the end of your walk, you won't really have seen a thing.

Let the magic portal of your attention open up to what is around you. Take a full breath, and begin your walk, with these goals in mind:

- **Walk quietly with open ears.** Listen for birds, breezes, movement, water. Try counting the number of sounds you hear. Once you start listening, it may feel like you notice the rich texture of the sounds of nature for the first time.
- **Notice the feel of the wind, your body as it moves, and your feet on the earth with each step.** As Thich Nhat Hanh says: "Print peace and serenity on the Earth. Walk as if you are kissing the Earth with your feet."[22]
- **Notice the changing views as you pass slowly.** Take in the ground, the plants, the sky, the colors, the light.
- **Pause to get close up, as close as you can.** Touch leaves, bark, flowers. Smell them. If you won't feel silly doing so, hug a tree trunk or at least lean against its weight and solidity.
- **Remind yourself you are made of nature.** The water in you is the water from this planet, your local groundwater

well or reservoirs. The pounds of microbiome you depend on (in your gut, lungs, skin) are shaped by your local environment, the produce you eat, the air you breathe (yes, there are millions of airborne microbes). Know and be known by the natural world, which you are part of.

When you walk in nature this way, with sensory portals open, the ruminative mind pauses, and whatever stress you are holding can dissipate, without your conscious effort. When you turn around to go home, you leave refreshed and ready to return to your demanding day with more reserves and a baseline set closer to green mind. You might take a photo of an image that moves you so you can re-experience this embodied feeling later.

Try bimbling for at least fifteen minutes—or as long as you can! Take an hour if possible. There is no such thing as "too much" nature immersion.

Option 2: Reset with Urban Nature

For the most effective urban getaway, find a place where you don't see or hear cars. You could go to a nearby park or waterfront, even a quiet neighborhood. This works best when you can be surrounded by trees or other greenery, have some kind of view, or be near water. But use what you have. There is always the sky.

The goal here is to use your senses and turn off your "city vigilance." If you can tap into your sensory experience here, you can get a helpful mini-version of the nature effect.

Take as much time as you have—even fifteen minutes can help your system reset. Walk slowly. Try to slow your breathing to your pace. Focus your attention on the elements of the natural world around you—see what you can notice. Observing wildlife, even in a cityscape, has an additional calming effect. You might see birds or squirrels. You can put up a feeder and attract hummingbirds to your yard. Watching a hummingbird, whose wings can beat up to eighty times per second, can induce feelings of awe.

Option 3: Bring Nature to You

For this method, bring nature into your own space. The senses are powerful. Sensations, smells, and sounds affect the nervous system. Studies on essential oils (from plants like cedar and especially lavender that release volatile organic compounds) show that inhalation leads to a brief but meaningful reduction in feelings of stress and anxiety.[23] This naturally works better with a short massage (rubbing it into your hands, feet, neck, or back). There are a lot of ideas out there about how essential oil aromas impact neurochemistry.[24]

Find a space in your home where you can be alone and can sit comfortably (either on a chair or on the floor) or lie down. If you have access to calming aromatherapy oils, use them. You can also bring nature objects inside—flowers, grass, leaves, acorns, anything that evokes the outdoors and the natural world. Activate auditory signals of nature.

Find an audio of nature sounds that resonate with you—wind, rain, waves (simply typing "nature sounds" on YouTube or a music streaming app gives generous choices). Then, do a short breathing activity to help nudge you into that "green to blue mind" state:

- Notice your flow of breathing, with one hand on your belly and one hand on your chest. You might feel your belly inflate more than your chest.
- Take five breaths through the nose, but breathe out more slowly than you breathe in.
- Now turn your focus outward, toward your senses and the room.
- Focus on any sounds. What does the air feel like as you breathe in? What do you smell? Do you want to feel or examine any nature objects?
- Imagine you are deep in a nature scene, whether it's by the water or in a forest, and visualize a detailed image.
- Tell yourself that this vast expanse of nature can hold any of your thoughts and emotions; it's big enough for all of your experience. Let it hold and support you right now.

However you decide to get your dose of nature, beauty, or awe, I'd like to leave you with a quote from John Muir: "Nature's peace will flow into you as sunshine flows into trees. The winds will blow their own freshness into you, and the storms their energy, while cares will drop off like autumn leaves."[25]

Troubleshooting

Not feeling the wonder that others are raving about? Some feel it easily and are quickly able to name it. Others just don't. You may not feel it in the way described, or it may not come to you readily. But that doesn't mean nature doesn't work for you. The natural world will still do its work on your nervous system, regardless.

There is no single recipe for awe, and it's not a requirement, no matter how gorgeous the landscape. You don't need to force it. There may be other types of experiences that bring you the sense of wonder and expansiveness that some people feel in front of a mountain range or the ocean. Watching videos of heroic human acts or space often induces feelings of awe. Awe is an experience we can cultivate with our attention and open curiosity about things we don't usually notice. Notice your surroundings, from tiny details to a full, zoomed-out view. You might try snapping five pictures each week of some sights that give you pause, and describe in a few words the emotions or thoughts they inspire.

If You Aren't Comfortable in Nature . . .

If being in raw, wild nature feels uncomfortable to you, take your time. An environment you perceive as unfamiliar or even threatening will rocket your vigilance in the wrong direction. This doesn't mean you can't tap into the power of nature. Try noticing plants and trees in your familiar neighborhood, or bringing the sounds and scents of nature into a space where you feel safe. Think about building up to more immersive nature experiences gradually.

You may have a strong preference for one type of nature over another. We have long known that people seek environments that fit their personality. Extroverts, for instance, have a higher need for social connection and activities, and feel more joy afterward than introverts, who will feel drained or taxed; extroverts feel comfortable in louder places like cafés. And, it turns out, they have their own, individual nature preferences: several studies by cultural psychologist Shigehiro Oishi and colleagues showed that extroverts prefer the ocean more than introverts do, whereas introverts prefer forests, mountains, and other quieter, more secluded places.[26]

Your personal preferences and comfort levels are worth respecting, but do try to push yourself a little bit. Novelty and exploration are also ways of expanding our resilience. Even if you feel a little "on alert" the first time in an unfamiliar ecosystem, my bet is you will quickly acclimate and begin to reap the stress-reducing rewards.

DAY 6

DON'T JUST RELAX ... RESTORE

FROM THE SECOND WE ARE BORN, WE BREATHE. BREATHING IS ESSEN-tial to our survival—yet the vast majority of us rarely take the time to think about our breath. Most of our breathing processes are involuntary, controlled by the brain stem. You breathe while you sleep. While you eat. While you talk. Of course, you can also choose to exert control over your breathing—we often notice and adjust our breath when we're exercising, for instance, or when we're getting upset, to calm ourselves down. But we are also influencing our breathing in other ways—ways we are not always aware of.

Several studies have found that when people are working, their breathing shifts. They breathe more times per minute; their breathing is more shallow. At work, we're breathing more rap-idly. There's even a phenomenon some call "email apnea": when you're checking email, you're likely to be holding your breath.

When we are holding tension—when the stress baseline is

high—we tend to take more breaths per minute, and those breaths tend to be shallow rather than deep. We respond to stress with light, rapid breathing, often through our mouth. A subtle pant! At the same time, this type of breathing *causes* a stress response in the body.[1] Shallow, fast breathing sends a signal to the body: get ready for action. That means a subtle version of fight or flight: vigilance in our nervous system. Our breath patterns—which are usually on autopilot and largely unconscious—both *influence* and *are influenced by* the stress and tension we are holding in the body. Ultimately this can become a kind of "stress spiral"—the stress of the day triggers a lighter, faster breathing pattern, marked by periods of unconscious breath holding, and that in turn keeps the body in a state of sympathetic nervous system activation. We end up in what we might call "orange mind"—breathing our way up into a state between cognitive load and stress arousal.

So let me ask you:

How much are you holding your breath?

How deeply or shallowly are you breathing?

How much tension are you holding in your body, in your chest?

Right now, at this moment, how much are you *fully* breathing?

The Problem: We Are Not Getting Real Rest

When you considered those questions above, what did you notice? Did you find that your shoulders were tensed? Your body or mind was leaning forward? Was your breathing slow and full, or light and shallow? Pause for a moment now and take a single, full breath—all the way in, all the way out—and consider: How does that feel compared with your typical breathing? Different?

This yellow mind state of constant nervous system activation, and the insufficient, light, fast breathing that goes with it, is just *normal* to us. We're used to it. We've accepted it as our baseline. So, when we face a period of higher stress, or a daily stressor that triggers a spike in our sympathetic nervous system, we ratchet up even higher—we go full red mind. When we come back down to our baseline of yellow mind, it feels like we've "relaxed." The problem is, we haven't. Or maybe more accurately: we have "relaxed" back to our default state. But our default state isn't relaxing enough.

It's not enough to come back down to baseline. We want to go *below* our habitual stress baseline—to true rest. Or, what I described earlier in this book as "deep rest" or "blue mind." When we can achieve this deep state of rest, it brings physiological restoration to the mind and body that we desperately need, and it helps us break out of this pattern of holding on to stress arousal.

When we can reach blue mind, even just for short periods, it not only leads to biological rejuvenation, but also has the potential to bring down our default stress baseline. As we discussed at the very beginning of this book, dropping our default stress baseline allows us to operate at a healthier and more biologically sustainable level of nervous system arousal.

We can't be in deep rest all the time—that's impossible. But do you know how often most of us are getting deep rest?

Almost never.

So today, I want to talk about deep rest. If we want to live a vibrant life with good stress resilience, deep rest is not optional. It's a requirement. It's as necessary as oxygen. And in fact, it has a lot to do with oxygen.

Constant states of high stress arousal mean shallow breathing and chronic wear and tear on our cells. This yellow mind stress state uses up our batteries faster. By the end of the day, we feel depleted; by the end of the week, we feel as if we aren't "recharging" at all. We need a break. We need to truly recharge and reset. We need to create conditions in which the body can perform some critical mind-, body-, and cell-rejuvenating processes that we have been skipping over. Our stress arousal level manifests in our breathing rate, as one of many factors shaping it. Spoiler alert: the deep rest we need is *also* about breathing.

When we are in deep rest, our breathing pattern becomes slow. More oxygen crosses the barrier between our lungs and our blood vessels. Nitric oxide levels rise, which causes blood vessels to dilate, letting blood and oxygen travel more quickly through the body. Blood pressure goes down; heart rate drops. These physiological processes are tightly linked to our breathing patterns. And all of these happenings in the body indicate that we are entering a blue mind state—a state of true, deep rest and relaxation.

So how do we get there?

Getting to Deep Rest—Harder Than It Seems!

You lounge on the couch, watching a show you love. You take your dog for walks or jogs. You cook your favorite meal, losing yourself in the smells and tactile processes of preparing food. You take a break from work to peruse social media and message with friends.

All of these activities sound deeply relaxing. Are they?

A mistake we all make is confusing breaks and leisure with true restoration. Taking breaks from work or caregiving and doing things you enjoy, like spending time with those you love, enjoying books and movies—this is all important! And yes, that is a form of relaxation: *green mind* category. But these do not bring you to deep restoration for two reasons. The first is that most likely, you still have a busy mind. Second, you *are* busy, and blue mind is most easily achieved when you are not doing, but being—when you are sitting or lying down, receptive, and focusing your attention on something other than your mental content. A lot of the things people do to relax are not truly restorative. They are valuable in their own right, but superficial compared with deep rest states. There is a big difference between green and blue mind.

Try to conjure up a time when you felt truly, completely relaxed. When you felt that your body and mind were getting a total break from work. Maybe you were in a particular place—a lot of people point to nature, because we saw from the previous chapter that nature can induce these types of blue mind states. Maybe it was more about where you *weren't*—you may have been away from the usual busy hubbub and demands of daily life. We don't typically reach states of deep relaxation while surrounded by piles of laundry to be folded, or the humming laptop with its promise of more emails. You also probably felt safe, because safety is a prerequisite of deep relaxation. Deep rest often overlaps with physical seclusion. There is a "sensory narrowing" or even deprivation—an absence of stimuli. We are in a receptive state of awareness (not leaning forward, poking ahead into the imagined future, but leaning back, or reclining flat). There is a sense of an open, gentle floating of the attention— we aren't worrying over anything in particular or getting caught up in rumination, but instead may feel daydreamy, creative, or drifty; we are able to calmly let thoughts arise and pass.

For some, when I ask them to call up a memory of deep relaxation, it's a vacation that comes to mind—a true escape. Some say a nature excursion. Others will cite a long massage. For me, it's the end of a long yoga class. Most yoga classes end with a pose called *Savasana*, or corpse pose, and the goal is to lie down on the ground, doing nothing, while the energetic resources of the body are recharged. At the end of Savasana, I reluctantly peel myself back up to get on with my day—but I do feel both calm and recharged. This state of deep relaxation is typical after mind-body practices like yoga, meditation, or qigong. If you've felt it, you've probably not wanted it to end! This is it: blue mind. A total break from busy mind activity, a period of wakefulness and alert restoration.

You may or may not have had much of this experience yet—

that's okay. Most of us have little of this per week or even year. Rest, it seems, should be the easiest thing to do—natural, effortless, automatic—but it's actually one of the most challenging. The idea of taking time out is hard, and the idea of "doing nothing" is even harder. As much as we might love to, we can't just plop down on the couch and quickly achieve deep rest. Our minds and bodies just don't downshift that quickly and easily. So it's certain activities like mind-body practices that really help us get there. Savasana is known within yoga to be the most important but most challenging pose to do well. This may seem strange, in a practice where some of the poses involve incredible feats of strength and flexibility! But the central tenet of the corpse pose is to *let go, to completely surrender control and truly relax*. There's a reason why Savasana comes at the very end of yoga practice: letting go is so hard for us that we need to prepare the mind and body to achieve it.

The Cellular Biology of Deep Rest

When deep rest happens, something unique occurs in the brain and body. It's the opposite of our default state of vigilance. Earlier this week, we talked about how the recovery process after hormetic stress creates a "cleanup process," activating scavengers that eat up free radicals and disposing of old parts and killing old cells. This cleanup process triggered by positive stress is excellent for your body at the cellular level. But deep rest does something different. Something more.

Deep rest causes biological restoration: it improves growth

hormone and sex hormones, and as these increase, the body is better able to restore, heal, and regenerate tissues. Having deep rest states while we are awake creates a potent form of restoration for our minds and bodies. During sleep, we have a deep rest phase as well: The stage of deep sleep (also called *slow-wave sleep*) is the most restorative state we have. There is a pulsing of cerebrospinal fluid, which cleans out amyloid proteins and other debris from our brain.

In the field of stress science, one of the ways we've measured the impact of deep rest has been to study people who go on retreats. *Retreat* can mean a lot of things. Often it refers to a structured meditation workshop or silent retreat, hosted at a retreat center, with trained facilitators. But that's just one end of the spectrum. *Retreat* in the true sense of the word can simply mean to remove yourself from your usual environment, the one filled with stimuli and demands. For example, staying alone in a cabin in the woods.

Retreat centers provide the ideal set of conditions that allow people to unwind more than usual. It's protected time; boundaries are enforced. You are safe; you are cut off from the things that often fire up your sympathetic nervous system (work, email, technology, caregiving demands, thorny relationships—whatever is going on out there in your usual milieu that may be triggering you into a state of activated arousal).

I know that, personally, I've felt the deepest states of rest during retreats, and the effects stay with me for weeks. In the long term, it's worth thinking ahead to how you might make room for a retreat of some kind—whether it's a formal program at a center or just a weekend away in the woods. Taking this kind of intensely protected, tech-free, rest-focused downtime for ourselves is something we rarely prioritize, but we need to. However, today, we don't have a week away from the swirl and whirl of our regular day-to-day. We have right now—while you're reading this chapter, and the few minutes you can carve out to try a new practice today. Can we create a "retreat" mindset in a much shorter period of time—something we don't need to take a week off work for, but can do *now*, and every day?

A "Retreat" State of Mind

The human brain, an organ isolated in the dark in the skull, is fully dependent on sensory inputs for current information. The brain works by then using all that information and predicting what might happen. Emotions are, most basically, the brain's best guess at how it should respond to a situation given the signals it's getting from the body, along with its memories of similar situations.[2] For example, if you've been dealing with numerous crises at work—answering one difficult email after another— the next time you hear the sound of an email landing in your inbox, you might find yourself slightly more tensed and vigilant before you even open the email. The brain's response is based on experience and habit. But we can break this cycle and shift our trajectory toward deeper rest states.

We can shape our brain activity and habitual states of stress arousal by changing the signals the brain is getting from the body. We can engineer a bodily experience that sends "corrective" signals to the brain, which shapes interoceptive cues, which in turn shapes how we feel right now. In other words, if we increase all the cues and conditions that tell our body we are safe, we are comfortable, there is nothing to do right now but relax, that's a strong formula to start with. We can use cues like dim light or darkness, soft pillows or eye masks, being in a certain safe and enclosed room, soothing images or symbols—these can all send the signal that it's okay to relax and let down our guard. In this state, the body eventually does the rest. It detects that it's in a safe environment to direct energy to housekeeping in our cells. And most important, this *feeds forward*. Experience in deep rest creates bodily memories. It will influence how the brain predicts the same sensory and interoceptive cues in the future. It's a positive feedback loop. We're adding new inputs that build deep rest into our future brain predictions. We will get to deep rest states more easily and quickly next time.

Retreats make deep rest easy. It would be lovely to create this "retreat" state of mind daily. I try to do this at night, during my wind-down ritual before sleep. If we look at the components of a successful retreat, you can create a similar experience wherever you are: You are disconnected from demands. Your phone is off—ideally, you don't even have the option to check it. You feel socially safe—you're either comfortably alone, in companionable silence, or with others who share this similar goal. In these conditions, the nervous system recalibrates. We disconnect from the sources of stress and reconnect to ourselves—to an inner core of calm. By taking away the demands of the outside world, we relieve our enormous cognitive load; through doing this for long periods, we also chip away at our stored-up unconscious stress.

What happens inside our cells when we're on retreat? This is the exact question my colleagues and I set out to investigate in a study we conducted in partnership with Drs. Rudy Tanzi and Eric Schadt.[3] Eric is a mathematician who, with sophisticated modeling, can identify patterns of change in the activity of over twenty thousand genes. For this study (the same study we discussed on Day 1), we recruited participants who had never meditated before—total newbies—and brought them all to a retreat center. We then split the group in half. One half received mantra meditation training that week, from Deepak Chopra and other teachers. The other half simply lived at the beautiful retreat center, ate the same healthy Ayurvedic meals, wandered the same lovely grounds. *Everyone* unplugged completely from work, phones, and computers.

It turned out that just living at the retreat center—regardless of whether the participants trained in meditation—created dramatic changes in gene expression activity in the immune cells, so much so that machine learning could predict the post-retreat profiles with 96 percent accuracy. Or put more simply—cell activity after living at the retreat center was dramatically different than it was on the day the participants arrived! We saw reductions in inflammatory activity, oxidative stress activity, DNA damage, and mitochondrial degradation. All great things! Autophagy-related processes—that beneficial process of cell cleanup—went up. People in both groups reported feeling full of vitality at the end of the week and had large decreases in depression, anxiety, and stress. The point is: you don't need to learn to meditate to experience health benefits. We simply put people in a beautiful relaxing environment (with no email), and it created rapid and powerful changes in the body.

The impact of mindfulness and meditation training can be profound. The stark contrast between the mind and nervous system of a person who is in the midst of an inwardly focused meditative practice and one who is immersed in a high-stress context is dramatic. The benefits are real. One young man who completed a mindfulness meditation class for refugees run by my colleague Professor Amit Bernstein described what it felt like: "It's a state of getting the mind rest and then after the mind gets rest you can bring a very clear, clean state of thinking. It's like a medicine for me. It might be a luxury for you, but it's a medicine for me. I use it like a medicine."[4]

The Right to Rest

We don't all have equal access to rest, based on our personal histories and structural factors. We all have our own unique challenges; we are all different, with intricately calibrated nervous systems, different triggers, different things that soothe us and make us feel safe. Thirty percent of us have experienced childhood trauma, which for most means feeling more threat from and vigilance toward daily stressors.[5] We also know now that people with early life trauma particularly benefit from mind-body practices that create deep rest.

Rest is a social justice issue—there are both socioeconomic and racial barriers to deep rest. We don't all have the same freedom and ability to get enough sleep. Groups targeted for marginalization, especially Black people in America, have rest inequity. Indeed, studies show that Black, Latinx, and Asian individuals in America have shorter and worse quality sleep compared with white Americans.[6] Tricia Hersey, a performance artist and community healer, founded the Nap Ministry based on the principle that rest is a form of resistance.[7] As she writes on her website: "We believe rest is a spiritual practice, a racial justice issue and a social justice issue."

Deep rest is a right, not a luxury. This is a societal and cultural shift that we are going to have to make, with science (and hard data!) leading the way. We collectively struggle with sleep because of the universal way the human mind works—it tends toward the yellow mind state of constant vigilance—and because of societal and work pressures on our time. Rest itself—true rest, deep rest—is powerful medicine, and it's scarce. We need to make it more accessible—for everyone. Beyond looking at the ways that you can make more space for yourself to rest, what sphere of wider influence might you have in your everyday life, where you can support others in getting the rest they need? This could be your immediate family circle, but it might also extend to friends, people who work for you, people with less privilege or opportunity. Are there ways you can advocate for rest?

You can feel how ingrained the anti-rest message is in you

just by noticing your reactions to the suggestion that you take time for deep rest. Reading this chapter, how many times did you catch yourself thinking, *I don't have time for rest*, or *I'm going to skip this chapter*, or *I can't rest; other people make it work with even more on their plate*, or *Maybe after I hit this deadline*. If you found yourself saying any of these things, *you need rest even more*.

This is about your health. Your life. It's about where you're heading, how you'll feel, and what your capacities will be once you get there. It's prevention, like brushing your teeth, which, you'll notice, you do manage to fit in every day. Countering stress every day is tending to our wellness, our quality of life, and our ability to make an impact in the world in some capacity— whatever our sphere of influence may be. *If you don't put in the time for self-care, including deep rest now, you'll be forced to make time for illness later.* Each day, we can create fertile ground for early aging and disease, or we can create the conditions for rejuvenation and wellness. Allow yourself to recharge.

Breathe Your Way to Deep Rest . . . Right Now

There's not one single way to create deep rest—there are a lot of ways to get there. You may get there during a long retreat. At the end of a workout. During Savasana at the close of a yoga session. Or being deep in nature, as our bodily processes fall in sync with the natural world. But there's one common change that happens with all those activities: a change in the breath to be more slow and rhythmic, and which leads to greater vagal tone (greater parasympathetic to sympathetic balance) and greater oxygen in the body.

When we create conditions that are ideal for deep rest—feeling safe, engaging in a mind-body practice, or being in nature—our breathing will often change naturally as the body adjusts. Today, we flip that. We *start* with the breath. When we practice the kind of breathing our body wants to do in a deep rest state, we signal to the body that it's okay to rest. It's okay to let go. Instead of a "top-down" way of creating a mental mindset of rest, like meditation, we use a "bottom-up" way: we change our mental and physical states through the breathing. Breathing, it turns out, can be the quickest, most direct path to deep rest. When you can't go to a retreat, you can bring the retreat to you. And all you need is your breath.

Breathing practices are one of the most powerful acts we can do to change our physiological state—and quickly. It's quite amazing: we can control our breath, which means we can control the state of our autonomic nervous system and even our state of consciousness. By altering our breath, we also influence our emotional state, pushing us toward calm, joy, and equanimity.

First: realize that you probably aren't breathing correctly most of the time! We spend most of our time breathing fast and inefficiently—a perfect recipe for orange mind, a higher-than-ideal stress baseline. We also breathe through the mouth too often. Breathing in through the nose allows our sinuses to create nitric oxide, which goes to our lungs and has a healthy vasodilatory effect. Journalist James Nestor, author of *Breath*, did his own personal research (me-search!) by taping his nose shut for ten days so he could breathe only through his mouth.[8] It demonstrated what he thought would happen, and worse—he felt anxious, his body was taken over by sympathetic dominance, his epinephrine shot up, and he did not sleep well. His snoring went from a few minutes a night to hours at night—and he even developed some sleep apnea. Returning to nose breathing resolved all of this.

A popular trend now is to use special tape to keep the mouth closed during sleep, such as Myotape, developed by breathing expert Patrick McKeown. After curing his own asthma, McKeown has devoted his career to showing others how changing the breath can help with many health issues.[9] Breathing physiology is complex and fascinating, but the actual practice of ideal functional breathing is—thank goodness—simple and graceful. Try the method in the box on the next page, which McKeown calls Light, Slow, and Deep (LSD) breathing. Don't take a big breath! Big breaths through the mouth create overbreathing, narrowing of vessels, and less oxygen in our blood. Light, gentle breathing leaves us with more oxygen in our blood! Does it feel different from how you normally breathe? The Breathe Light, Slow, and Deep exercise involves working with a tolerable feeling of air hunger to increase CO_2 in the lungs and the blood, and slowing the breath down. At first, the feeling of air hunger may be uncomfortable, but as your tolerance to CO_2 increases, you will find it easier.

McKeown advises trying this gently at first, in thirty-second bursts with a one-minute rest in between. He suggests starting with light breathing for air hunger, then adding the expansion and contraction of the lower ribs, and finally, slowing down the breath while keeping the breathing volume minimal. All together, this normalizes breathing biochemistry, biomechanics, and rate. Light, slow, nasal, and diaphragmatic breathing form the basis of functional everyday breathing.

This is how we should be breathing, as much as possible.

BREATHE WELL

Sit up straight to leave your air passageways open and clear: chest up, chin down. Breathe with your mouth closed, through your nose. Breath easily and comfortably, using the *light, slow, deep* method:

Breathe **lightly**—softly, gently, quietly

Breathe **slowly**

Breathe **deeply**—down into your diaphragm (ribs widening to the sides)

Most of us are not aware of how much control we wield over our nervous systems through our breath. By simply altering our breathing rate, we can manipulate the oxygen and CO_2 levels in our lungs, blood, and tissues. For millennia, people have used breathing practices to energize, relax, and even create ecstatic states. There's an incredible spectrum of physiological and mental states you can create through breath. Yes, it can relax you. It can also increase hormetic stress (as in the Wim Hof method described earlier), taking you to a peak stress response—completely through breathing patterns. There are other breath practices, like holotropic breathing or, in yoga, kundalini breathing, which can dramatically change your level of consciousness and emotional states. We can use breathing to feel everything from stress to bliss to deep relaxation.

Our breathing practice today, which we'll start in just a moment, is going to involve some brief *breath holding*. Why? Because when we hold our breath, even briefly, we increase the amount of CO_2 in our blood. This allows hemoglobin, which carries oxygen, to release that oxygen into our blood and into our tissues. In short: it increases the amount of oxygen available to our body and brain briefly, until it's used up. Higher oxygen levels can be both energizing *and* relaxing, decreasing stress and increasing calm, clarity, and focus. And it turns out that brief breath holding can increase our "CO_2 tolerance level." The more CO_2 tolerance we have, the less anxiety we feel. We will do a brief breath hold in our practice today.

Studies of slow breathing exercises, in which participants are guided to exhale longer than they inhale, show that this can change the autonomic nervous system almost *immediately*.[10] As you slow down your breathing, the rest of your body falls in line: Slower heart rate. Increased brain alpha waves. General feelings of well-being and relaxation. And higher heart rate variability, which is significant because when we increase our heart rate variability (also called "vagal tone"), we send messages to our brain that we are safe. We give a break to our overworked sympathetic nervous system and reduce our cells' metabolic rate, allowing cellular rejuvenation. Across studies, slow breathing at a rate of ten breaths or less per minute, several times a week for a month, for about fifteen minutes per session (the exact length varies by the study), was shown to reduce systolic blood pressure by around six points. Researchers generally agree that slower is better—when we reduce our breathing to six breaths per minute, we can more reliably increase our heart rate variability and reduce blood pressure. This is called *resonant breathing* or *vagal breathing.*

Our normal respiration rate is twelve to twenty breaths per minute, with an average of around sixteen. Some of us even hover along the edge of hyperventilation. At our usual yellow mind default state of stress, our breathing is too fast and too shallow. And when we breathe fast and shallow, the body reacts with a stress response; it's a vicious cycle.

We all tend toward yellow mind, or an elevated baseline. It's a reflection of our good survival wiring: our attention is more biased toward threats, as they are exponentially more salient than the subtle signals of safety and love. It takes intention and creating a safe container to bring ourselves below our typical baseline for any extended period. That entails more work than it takes for us to react to stress, which is automatic. Deep rest states take conscious effort at first, and time.

So today, I'd like you to try to slow your breathing rate down, whenever you can. And in our practice, we're going to learn a specific technique for slow and restorative breathing. This is a tool that you can—and should!—use anytime you need a nervous system reset. It probably won't get you to a deep rest state without adjusting some of the other parameters I'm going to give you for this practice, but it will break through chronic nervous system activation. Your breath is something you always have access to as a powerful form of stress relief.

Let's Recap

When we take shallow, quick breaths, we send stress signals to the body.

When we make long exhalations, we send signals to the body that we are safe. Parasympathetic nervous system activity increases; heart rate variability goes up (a good thing). Vagal tone improves.

Changing our breathing can change the mind. It can change the body's state of stress arousal. It can wash away anxiety and leave us relaxed, positive, resilient.

Relaxation is not enough; it doesn't meaningfully change our default stress baseline. And our default baseline is likely closer to *stress* than to *rest*. That means we are carrying around stress constantly. We are never dipping down into the blue mind state of true restoration that we need. To move the baseline, we need periods of restoration. Prolonged restoration is great. But even brief periods of restoration can be very powerful. A "mini-retreat" today goes a long way.

So let's breathe our way there now.

BREATHE YOUR WAY TO DEEP REST

Go-Bag Skill: Access Deep Rest States

This practice has a few prerequisites. Deep rest doesn't happen when we are connected to email, or anticipating texts or phone calls. It doesn't happen in places where we feel unsafe or uneasy. It requires seclusion, feeling safe, and being disconnected from daily demands. So step one is to prepare your space and connect with your body. As Thich Nhat Hanh says, "Breathe in deeply to bring your mind home to your body."

Prepare Your Space

Create the container! Choose a place you feel the most safe and relaxed. This spot is where you are most likely to have privacy and be away from work, chores, or other demands. Wherever you choose should be relatively quiet and clear of clutter.

You're going to lie down, so grab a yoga mat or blanket—whatever will make you comfortable. If you have an eye mask, weighted blanket, or pillows you can use as neck or knee supports, gather those. But know that you can do this without any props at all. One busy parent I know goes into the bathroom (the only space where no one will bother her!) and tosses a large towel on the floor.

Breathing for Restoration (4-6-8)

Recall the "breathe well" method of slower, deeper, more intentional breathing we tried earlier in the chapter. Flip back to the box on page 159 if you need a refresher. That's what we want to do all day, when we remember to slow our breath down. For a short breathing exercise, we are now going deeper, into a practice that is aimed at absorbing your full attention, to increase your vagal tone and oxygenation.

Set a timer for five minutes (I suggest taking the time to select a gentle tone or song to alert you when the time is up). Lie down on your mat or blanket, using support pillows to get comfortable, if you like. Close your eyes. You might mentally put down that suitcase of bricks (from Day 2). Now, for the next five minutes:

- Breathe in for four seconds through the nose.
- Hold for six seconds
- Breathe out very slowly for eight seconds. Try exhaling through pursed lips to slow your breath if that feels easier.

In for four, hold for six, out for eight: Repeat this pattern, trying to breathe deep into your diaphragm and imagining your breath radiating through your body, to the tips of your fingers and the ends of your toes.

For many people, even just a few minutes of this deep relaxation breathing will profoundly affect the nervous system, doing a kind of "reset." My hope is that you will return to your day recalibrated, grounded, and with less yellow mind going forward. But don't write it off if you don't see immediate effects the very first day. The impact of a practice like this increases over time. If this feels uncomfortable, start with 4-4-6 (breathe in for four, hold for four, and breathe out for six). Use gentle breaths. Don't give up!

Bonus Practice

Five Percent More with Mindfulness

If you have a little more time today, tack on an extra five to ten minutes after your breathing practice for a short mindfulness check-in. Research has shown that even brief regular sessions of mindfulness practice can improve attention and bring down stress. It can also offer you profound insights into what stressors you are holding in your mind and in your body.

Mindfulness is, in a nutshell, paying attention to our momentary experience without judgment, and with kindness. This is simple, but not easy! So do this with 100 percent commitment and 100 percent forgiveness. There is no way to do this "badly." Our body breathes by itself, so all we have to do is observe this process, and it can be a rich and relaxing experience.

Place attention on your breath. (Don't worry about counting anymore—just breathe naturally.) Notice the breath-related sensations in your body as the air goes in and out. When your mind wanders away, to worries or thoughts, move your attention back to the breath and the sensations in your body.

Check in with your body:

- What sensations and energy level do you feel? Can you sense your body's quiet energy? It may feel like humming, buzzing, or vibrations. Where are you still holding stress? Remember the "catch and release" exercise we started the week with? That fits in right here: As you breathe, scan your body for stored stress, and let it go. Notice any feelings of ease.
- As you breathe in, think of the word *refresh*. Breathe out, and think, *Relax*. Or visualize a colorful circle or mandala expanding and shrinking with each inhale and exhale. **Can you let your nervous system relax just 5 percent more?**

And finally, if you can, leave your relaxation space set up for tomorrow, and plan to do this practice again around the same time. Our body can be conditioned to relax more automatically! Let's take advantage of that. Doing this practice around the same time, in the same space, and with a sensory trigger (aromatherapy scents or soothing sounds) will, with time and repetition, condition your body to move more quickly into a state of rest and rejuvenation.

Troubleshooting

If Changing Your Breathing Made You Feel Anxious . . .

If you look closely at studies on breathing, you learn that for many of us, when we jump into new methods of slow breathing, we develop subtle hyperventilation (dizziness, tingling, tension) caused by decreases instead of increases in blood CO_2. That means we may feel more anxious than relaxed. This is particularly true for people with asthma or anxiety. There's a quick fix, and I know it sounds counterintuitive: *Breathe shallowly (lightly), naturally, and slowly. Avoid deep breathing.* Just those instructions helped people immediately benefit from the vagal breathing.[11]

Some of you might have high levels of anxiety sensitivity, sometimes called *fear of fear*—this is an intolerance of the physical symptoms of anxiety. For example, feeling your own heart beat fast might make you even more anxious. During COVID, we saw that having high anxiety sensitivity predicted both development of more severe anxiety and depression, as well as more visits to the doctor.[12] If you have high anxiety sensitivity, you especially need to retrain yourself to breathe longer and slower breaths. In extreme cases, for people with panic disorder, changing their breathing in this way, toward hypoventilation, can even reduce panic attacks.[13]

In studies of breathing retraining, people sometimes get worse before they get better. For example, in studies of slow, resonant breathing (six breaths per minute), people—especially those with high anxiety—have more signs of hyperventilation when they first start the retraining. They feel more relaxed after a few weeks. So start slow, stick with it, and know that you might feel worse before you feel better, but it will be worth it.

DAY 7

START FULL, END FULL

WHAT'S THE FIRST THING YOU THINK ABOUT WHEN YOUR EYES OPEN IN the morning?

Do you wake up to a beeping alarm and immediately start thinking, *What time is it? Am I late?* Do you roll over and pick up your phone? Do you wake to the sound of a child or pet calling for you? Are you already thinking about the logistics of the day, and how you're going to get everything done?

Waking up, we'd love to greet the new day as a clean slate. A fresh start, a blank white page of possibility. But it's not. We have all kinds of worries to deal with—leftovers from yesterday, and fresh ones for today.

But how we wake up, those first few precious minutes after our eyes fly open (or creak reluctantly open, in some cases), has a huge influence over the rest of our day—and, in fact, over our stress resilience and our physiology. So does how we end the day. Think of these two short spans of time like bookends—first thing in the morning and last thing at night—that frame and contain your daily experience. These brief moments are crucial to how you calibrate yourself to the coming day before it happens, and then how you wind down and reflect on your day— what you choose to focus on and highlight—at the end of it.

How you wake up to greet the day calibrates your reactivity to stressors. How you wind down shapes your sleep and restoration. These choices at the beginning and end of your day may affect the functioning of your mitochondria—the "batteries" of your cells. These choices can lead to days when you feel more joy. And *joy* is what we're talking about today, because the more of it you can have in the course of a day, the less stress you'll feel.

Doses of Joy

We know that when we experience more joy—not fleeting pleasure, but what we call *eudaemonia,* or "happiness with purpose," we are more stress resilient for a simple reason: we just don't feel as much stress. We don't have to work as hard on how we respond to it, or how quickly we recover. We simply don't register it in the first place. We have become immune.

At the very beginning of this book, we talked about how much of our stress stems from uncertainty. From fear of what might happen, of the unknown, of all the ways our best-laid plans can go awry. Another way to look at this is that much of our stress stems from our love. We experience stress because we care. We are driven by love—the other major force in our life, next to fear. We feel stress and worry because we care about the people we love. We care about doing well in our work. We care about the country we live in, the planet we live on. We care so much, and so much can go wrong, that it's easy to feel like we're sinking—like our stress is too big, too much, too overwhelming.

Chade-Meng Tan, a former software engineer and Google pioneer, has a beautiful analogy for this: We go through life as if we're in a little boat. Our boat is out in the ocean, traveling over the waves. And it floats! It only sinks when water gets in. If your little boat is sinking, the problem isn't the water itself. Water simply exists. The problem is that it's gotten *in*.

We are all surrounded by this ocean of stress and pain. And that's always going to be there. We can't drain this ocean away. But we don't have to. The problem isn't the ocean. The problem happens when the ocean water gets in. So how can we be resilient? How can we keep the water out and stay afloat?

It's a big question. Some days can feel hard—like we're bailing that little boat out all day long, and barely keeping afloat. Ultimately there are many factors that are at play when it comes to how resilient we are as individuals. Some of them are beyond our control, like genetics, our past experiences and how they have shaped us, our socioeconomic circumstances, and more. Others we can work on, like our mindset and where we put our attention. We've seen evidence throughout this book for how certain interventions can change our stress response and help us float better, with more ease. But the research shows us that when it comes to building stress resilience, one of the most powerful interventions is focusing on joy—specifically, the positive things that exist in our lives now, and on creating a positive future.

It's simple, but the science backs it up: joy will float your boat.

Today is our last day together. And I hope it's the most fun. Joy is the focus today, and we're going to achieve it in a couple of ways. We're going to talk about the things, both large and small, that create real happiness and life satisfaction, the kind that is stress buffering, the kind that really makes our boat float. I'm going to share some small things you can easily fold into your day to boost joy—little actions that go a long way. And our practice is going to focus on the bookends of our day—the first few minutes after you wake up, and the last few minutes before you fall asleep.

Think of these like pressure points of the day—if you know just where to apply a little bit of effort, your whole nervous system will respond.

"Stress Habits" and Happiness

When someone participates in one of our lab's stress studies, we text them twice a day with surveys they fill out on their phones: once in the morning, and again at night. We want to capture their first waking thoughts, and their last before drifting off.

The questions in the morning look like:

- How much are you looking forward to today?
- How much are you dreading today?
- How much joy or contentment do you feel?
- How worried, anxious, or stressed do you feel?

And at the end of the day, we ping them again.

- What was the most stressful thing that happened to you today?
- How much did you think about it afterward? For how long?
- What was the most positive thing that happened today?
- Did you tell anyone about a good thing that happened to you?

The data my team and I get from these surveys is so rich. The answers to these questions reveal people's *stress habits*. We call them stress habits because while each day differs, especially when it comes to random events that occur, it turns out that we each have a habitual style of thinking: if we wake up feeling positive on one day, it's likely we do on most days.

When we blend these self-reported survey results with the objective physiological data from the lab, we can see how some people are able to create more positive emotion that buoys them through the stress of their day. Research on daily mood, especially after a hard day, shows that low levels of positive emotions (or high negative emotions) predict poor long-term health, like depression, heart disease, even mortality.[1] In another study, those who maintained a positive outlook after a lab stressor had less inflammation and were less likely to have depression in the following year.[2] This is the same positive response to stress we discussed in Day 3—feeling challenge, confidence, and hope.

When we feel positive emotions (across the spectrum, from satisfaction and contentment to social connection to sensory pleasure), it immediately gives us a break from stress. Similar to going out into a deep green forest or practicing slow breathing, happiness has a physiological effect on the body. Happiness tempers stress, making its effects less potent. [3] This is especially true for people coping with a chronic illness, when it's easy to let stress overshadow the positive things in life.

Happiness also has a measurable impact on cognition. In other words, it shapes the way your brain functions—in particular, your attention. Positive emotions (joy, happiness, contentment, ease) work as an antidote to that kind of ruminative narrowing of focus that our human minds have a tendency to do. Joy and happiness broaden our attention and boost adaptive coping, which is our mental capacity to reframe problems rather than rigidly fixate on them. [4] Reframing—focusing on the silver lining in a bad situation—takes some mental work. It requires cognitive bandwidth to accomplish. You might go from feeling upset about another pandemic cancellation, for example, to thinking to yourself, *Well, I have been wanting more time with my kids, and now I have it—they're growing up so fast.* People who report more general happiness tend to have *more* of that broad attention and mental space to make those kinds of pivots—which then can boost satisfaction and neutralize stress even more. And positive, happy emotions reduce our emotional reactivity to the next stressful thing that occurs. [5] And we enjoy other cognitive benefits: We can be more creative. We solve problems better. We connect with other people more easily. [6]

There are even physical health effects from having a positive mindset: it's anti-inflammatory, buffering the effects of stress so that even people who've experienced high levels of adversity in life are less likely to develop high systemic inflammation.[7] Higher levels of positive emotion can even predict protection from the common cold: it's good for your immunity![8] A meta-analysis that controlled for health and other factors found that it's also correlated with increased longevity.[9] The more positive emotions you tend to feel, the longer you may live.

The science on happiness and joy is pretty clear: it's good for the mind, good for the body, good for stress resilience. So how do we get more of that?

You Can't Chase Happiness

What has been the most popular college class at Yale? Happiness. Berkeley? Happiness. Harvard? Happiness. The topic masquerades with different names and variations, but all focus on components of happiness. At Michigan, it's purpose. What about at Stanford? The most popular class historically has been on . . . stress! The actual title is Behavioral Biology, and it has been taught by the stress research pioneer Dr. Robert Sapolsky. This is the class that turned me toward seeking a life of inquiry to better understand suffering and love, and how to live well. There, we students learned that we are really not that different from monkeys in clothes—we are driven by survival instincts run by our nervous system, hormones, neurotransmitters, and other invisible influences, more than we know or want to know—but also that we can transcend our biology and live meaningful spiritual lives.

But here's a paradox for you: happiness is a wonderful salve for stress, but you can't go out there seeking it. If you say, "My goal is to be happy," then, the research shows, you are actually more likely to achieve the opposite. Tal Ben-Shahar, who teaches the Harvard class, describing the fallacy of the pursuit of happiness, puts it this way: "You cannot look directly at the sun, but you can absorb its rays." It's ironic, because in the US, the "pursuit of happiness" is baked into the language in our Declaration of Independence. But surveys reveal that people who actively pursue happiness, overvalue the idea of happiness, or believe they should be happy most of the time are some of the unhappiest people.

Positive emotions *are* powerful. But we can't seek happiness directly. We have to know what factors actually create it.

Dr. Ben-Shahar refers to the ingredients for happiness with an acronym, SPIRE, which stands for spirituality, physical activity, intellectual activity, high-quality relationships (in other words, deep, not superficial), and positive emotional experiences. These ingredients for happiness stretch across many arenas of your life, and we can't tackle everything here in just one day. But I bring this up to remind us of where lasting happiness actually comes from—because that helps us to identify the elements that are already in our day-to-day lives that we might be missing and want to amplify. Instead of chasing an abstract idea of "happiness," we can intentionally place ourselves in these SPIRE experiences, building the infrastructure of long-term happiness into our future. And when we can focus our attention on the ways we *already have* some of these experiences, we magnify our feelings of contentment. Contentment is a durable and solid form of happiness, and it's often more accessible. The happiness of *contentment* is always possible.

Joy Is an Inside Job

True joy isn't something we can buy or acquire—it comes from within. This may be hard to believe if you've been raised in a Western culture, because it's the opposite of all the social and media conditioning we've received.

A few years ago, I had the opportunity to participate in a group leading stress resilience retreats as part of the World Economic Forum, in Davos, Switzerland. This is the annual meeting of global financial conglomerates where there are high-profile public talks, but also a lot of backroom meetings where acquisitions and mergers and other plans that affect the global economy are being discussed. Up in a quiet ski lodge with crisp panoramic views of the Alps, a far cry from the frantic conference center, we listened to Tibetan Buddhist teacher Tsoknyi Rinpoche lead a section on genuine happiness. Rinpoche shared that true happiness is not achievable through material acquisition and achievements but rather is already right here (as he said *here*, he pointed to his heart). It is within each person, ready to be more fully discovered and brought out.

In the audience, a man's hand shot up. He shook his head vigorously and said, "No, no, no. We're achievement oriented.

We get fulfillment from reaching goals, and we really do like material acquisitions, that's what brings us happiness."

There was some nodding, a few heads were shaking, but across the board, everyone's attention was at a pinpoint. The room hushed. The elephant in the room had been named.

Rinpoche smiled, delighted. He walked closer to the man who had asked the question. I was riveted: the CEO in the black suit, face-to-face with the monk in the red robes.

"I saw an ad for a new iPad," Rinpoche said. "In this ad, the man holding the iPad was so attractive and youthful and strong. He had a washboard stomach and I wanted to be like him. So I bought the iPad. It felt so good to hold it. I felt like my stomach was made of muscle. But then I looked down and my belly was round and soft!"

He rubbed his stomach and smiled. Everybody laughed, disarmed.

"And then my iPad broke down. Now my shiny new iPad is damaged and my happiness is gone."

It was a simple story, almost a parable, but Rinpoche went on to talk more deeply about the issue of hooking happiness to material goods or even specific goals. Mastery and goal achievement can make us feel good temporarily. And it can be part of the road to happiness and life purpose. But we have to also see the big picture. We cannot always be chasing what is better, thinking that if we just get this amount of money, or acquire this item (an iPad, a house, a car, even a job), we'll be happy. There's always a new thing. A better thing. A bigger thing. Someone more accomplished than us.

There's always another goal, beyond the one
As we said earlier this week, we can't allow our
dependent on things in the outside world that
trol. We can be ambitious and achievement or
hanging too much of our happiness and self-worth on to the next
thing we are trying to get or do. And surprisingly, one of the best
ways to be happy is to embrace our negative or difficult emotions
and be okay with them.

Tsoknyi Rinpoche led everyone in a meditation called the
"handshake with emotion."[10] The instruction was to recall a recent experience that was emotionally stressful, and to relive it
through memory, noticing how it feels in the body. Then, instead of trying to push away those negative emotions, you explore them in a gentle and spacious way, meeting and welcoming
whatever arises. Rinpoche calls them "friendly monsters" because these thorny visitors offer insight and wisdom. As you
open up to and identify negative emotions, you can soften
around them; you might even embrace or thank them. In neuroscience, we have a similar but simpler practice called *affect
labeling*, in which we ask you to describe in words what you
might be feeling right now. *Fear. Embarrassment. Jealousy.*
When we don't resist, fight, or run from negative emotions, but
instead face and embrace them, we dissolve their activating
power. We go from red mind to yellow mind, and eventually to
green mind as these negative emotions fade away. Plus, the research shows that the more types of *different* emotions we feel
and name, the more stress resilient we are and the lower our inflammation.[11] Like biodiversity, emotional diversity may indicate

an adaptable ecosystem. Naming emotions helps us increase that diversity.

The point here is that when it comes to well-being, chasing material pleasure doesn't work. Running from pain and stress doesn't work. What does work: noticing contentment and joy.

Balancing *Pleasure* and *Happiness*

Both pleasure and happiness are important to our well-being, but pleasure is short-lived. We often get it from consuming things (food, sex, consumer goods), which delivers a dopamine hit . . . and which feels *good*. That dopamine hit reinforces our desire to seek out that experience again—which isn't always the best thing for our long-term happiness, because the pleasure of consumption isn't lasting. We quickly experience a drop back down to our typical levels of happiness even after a major happy event. On the flip side, we can also rebound from a tragic event fairly quickly. We call this *hedonic adaptation*. We've even seen that lottery winners who have millions of dollars drop into their lap, and people who suddenly become paraplegic, both return to their baseline of happiness after a couple of years.

To be clear: there is nothing wrong with pleasure! Sensory pleasures—taking a scented bath, savoring delicious food, enjoying a massage, listening to music—are an integral part of the rich tapestry of human life . . . *and* they reduce stress as well. Being mentally present in a moment of sensory enjoyment is a wonderful way to recalibrate the nervous system. Another potent example is sex, which is one of the most amazing ways ᴜ. brains are wired for pleasure. The research on sexual activity shows that it tends to be related to better cardiovascular health and is stress buffering. Oxytocin, the "love hormone" that is released during orgasm or physical intimacy, reduces blood pressure, for example. And in our study on caregiving parents, we found that couples who had more frequent sexual intimacy tended to have longer telomeres and better metabolic health.

While it still remains somewhat of a taboo topic, sexual activity, whether dyadic (with a partner) or alone, is an important health behavior that should be on the list of quick ways to reduce stress. One study of couples found that feeling greater sexual satisfaction was linked to lower stress levels,[12] and in a survey of German[13] women that polled the group about their motivations for masturbating, 67 percent said they self-pleasure for relaxation and stress reduction. It was almost as common a reason as for pure sexual satisfaction itself (69 percent).

It's not necessarily just the act of sex itself that causes stress reduction—it's what the famed psychotherapist and relationship expert Esther Perel calls "erotic sensuality." She describes how erotic sensory experiences start with ourselves: "Erotic self-care begins with diminishing our inner-critic and giving ourselves simply the permission to feel beautiful, to enjoy our own company, to be more compassionate and realistic with ourselves."[14] All kinds of attention-captivating, immersive, and pleasurable sensory experiences bring some type of joy—subtle or strong, calm or ecstatic. The taste of, say, a delicious chocolate chip cookie fresh from the oven. The soft sensations of a breeze on your skin as you sit outside on a summer night. A relaxing, long, hot shower. The more we pause in these moments, keep our attention on them, appreciate them, experience them, the more joy we feel—and that's a stress melter.

We absolutely should encourage ourselves to appreciate and savor these moments of sensory delight, of being deeply in the body, of enjoying the moment. And at the same time, we should remind ourselves that hedonic pleasure—pleasure that is achieved through experiences of enjoyment from consuming or acquiring—is fleeting and impermanent, and that seeking it constantly isn't going to bring us the more lasting feelings of satisfaction and fulfillment that are the foundation of true happiness. In fact, excess pleasure seeking actually makes us miserable, and it is the basis for many of our addictions.[15] It puts us on a roller coaster—we may have *high* highs, but these are inevitably followed by *low* lows.

Getting off the Roller Coaster

New research that looks closely at the dynamics of emotion reveals that a stable mood is healthier than having dramatic fluctuations in positive emotion. Even if you have a lot of "high highs," it turns out that the more ups and downs you experience in positive emotion throughout the day, the more you suffer, with worse mental health[16] and lower vagal tone.[17] Routinely swinging up and down in positive mood is even linked to earlier mortality.[18]

So we are not aiming for the big peaks here! With peaks come valleys, and the up-and-down is simply a rough way to live. What we're aiming for is sustainable yet high enough positive emotion, and this comes from more stable sources of joy: feelings of satisfaction, contentment, and equanimity—these, the science shows, are extremely robust in counteracting daily stress.

Our goal here is "eudaimonic well-being," which has to do with feeling content, satisfied with life, and filled with purpose. It's rooted in your relationships with and connections to other people, and the most important thing about it is that it is *lasting*. While hedonic happiness—happiness that is achieved through experiences of pleasure and enjoyment—is fueled by bursts of dopamine transmission, eudaimonic happiness is regulated by serotonin.[19] Eudaimonic happiness is durable. It isn't vulnerable to the sometimes wild ups and downs of hedonic pleasure.

We all want to feel good. It's the stable, *low*-arousal positive emotion that that we want to cultivate. That's what is attainable and sustainable . . . and best for the mind and body.

Sounds great. So where do we get it?

There are many different paths to sustainable happiness. I am part of a National Institutes of Health research network on emotional well-being, and our first job was to come to a definition we could all agree upon. This was no easy task, and my colleagues who are deep experts in well-being took many months to agree on a single definition. The group finally converged upon something along these lines, although it is still evolving: Emotional well-being is complex, encompassing how we feel generally, in the moment, and about life overall. It has both *experiential* features, such as the emotional quality of our everyday experiences, and *reflective* features—our views about life satisfaction, social connections, and sense of meaning, and our ability to pursue goals that can extend beyond the self. So feelings of joy are just one component of overall well-being, but an important building block.

Enhancing any one of the ingredients below improves our well-being:

• Noticing moments of contentment, joy, or appreciation
• Having positive social connections
• Waking up feeling a sense of purpose about our day

I want to make an important point here: feelings of joy are accessible to everyone—no matter our circumstances. Remember my friend Bryan, whom we met at the beginning of this book? As a young man, he had been conscripted into the Russian army and sent off to one of the most unforgiving, inhospitable landscapes on our planet. He was pulled away from his family and put into what became, every day, a survival situation. He worried that he wouldn't see his loved ones again. He was constantly bothered by the extreme cold, by the grueling hours, by the menial labor he was tasked to perform.

But when he radically accepted that there were simply things he couldn't control about his situation, he was able to cope better. He let go of trying to fight against what he couldn't change, and he learned a valuable lesson about where he should put his energies, and how to be resilient and steady through tough times. Now, when unexpected, stressful, or scary things happen, he doesn't throw himself against a brick wall trying to change the things he can't change. He knows when to push for change, and when to adapt and accept. It's a valuable skill, something I marvel at—he's so good at it! But the thing that really strikes me about Bryan is his capacity for joy—even in the most uncertain, high-stress times. He seems to have unlimited access to it. He tells me that once he accepted his situation, all those years ago during his long deployment, he was able to find moments of elation. Even small things that never used to delight him began to bring him great joy. On his single day off every week, he would go on a walk and feel sheer bliss to just be able to do as he pleased—something he'd always taken for granted before. He could go into a little market, browse the food, buy anything he wanted, and revel in the flavors. He could stop and talk to someone he met in the street—even a brief chat about the weather—and he would feel like he was absolutely soaring, just to have a casual conversation with a kind stranger. After the long week of rigid schedules, sensory deprivation, and harsh conditions, every small pleasure seemed amplified—louder, brighter, more beautiful.

Bryan has a comfortable life now in San Francisco—no more survival gear on the arctic tundra for him. But he has retained this capacity to amplify the small pleasures in his life—he appreciates moments and experiences that might otherwise simply pass him by. He now knows that they are precious. And they are *fuel*.

pretend that we've all been dealt an equal hand in
certainly haven't. Some have had to journey along a
her road than others. Still, there is always *some*
beauty on that road. And it's true that some people will walk
down the smoothest road with the most stunning views and
notice only the pothole they have to step over, while others can
tackle a rough and rocky uphill slog and come away immensely
pleased about a single flower they found blooming between the
rocks. The more we can be like the latter person, the more resilient we will be—and the science supports this.

The actor Jim Carrey once said, "I think everybody should
get rich and famous and do everything they ever dreamed of so
they can see it's not the answer." Fame and wealth don't automatically bring happiness—but many people continue to live
their lives in hot pursuit of both. Culturally, there's a gulf between what we believe will bring us happiness and what really
does. Basic needs must be met for health and security. But once
our basic needs are met, studies show that higher incomes are
not associated with increased happiness.

We simply cannot buy joy. But we can find it, every day.

Capturing Joy: It's the Little Things

Dr. Sonja Lyubomirsky of the University of California, River-
side, one of the earliest pioneers in this field, has been conduct-
ing experiments on happiness for three decades. One of the
conclusions of her research is that while some of our "happiness
level" is determined by genetic factors and life circumstances,

a large portion is under our control.[20] Her research shows that people can measurably improve happiness and well-being through their intentional, daily behaviors—and maintain that boost long term. The further good news is that we don't necessarily have to make big, earthshaking changes to our lives to find more joy—little things can make a difference. One of the best ways to boost happiness is through small acts of kindness and compassion. One study tested the effects of doing something kind for others as opposed to doing something kind for ourselves, and it was the prosocial acts—doing something kind for others—that reduced stress and increased positive emotion.[21] Building on that, Lyubormirsky found that acts of kindness are linked to lower inflammatory gene expression.[22] Doing something kind for another person is good for them, good for your stress, *and* good for your body.

Relationships are important for health and happiness—in fact, strong relationships with partners, family, or friends are one of the most important factors in stable eudaimonic happiness. It's the positive emotions exchanged during relationships that are part of the magic. Researchers examined how couples dealt with conflict in the lab, and found that during conflict, those who *share* positive emotions at the same moments have nervous system reactivity profiles that are synced up. And the more they show this profile of syncing, the higher the quality of their relationships and the better their health, even years later.[23] Good relationships consistently predict health and happiness: people with higher-quality friend, family, or marital relationships tend to have better health and longevity.[24]

Positive emotion is powerful, and sometimes it's the small interactions in relationships that matter most. Even fleeting, passing interactions with a stranger can give you a powerful zing of positivity. Smiles can be a source of joy! A genuine full smile is like throwing a little party in the brain—your brain responds to your face muscles smiling by releasing feel-good chemicals like endorphins. Just like breathing can influence your nervous system from the "bottom up," so can a smile—smiling can make us feel a little happier.[25] It's called the *facial feedback hypothesis*. As Thich Nhat Hanh says, "Sometimes your joy is the source of your smile, but sometimes your smile can be the source of your joy."

Just as our breathing can shape our nervous system activity, just as a smile can shape our emotions, our mornings—in fact, the very first minutes after we open our eyes—can shape our whole day. Especially when it comes to how stress resilient we are.

Morning and Your Mitochondria

At the beginning of this chapter, I asked you to reflect on what you think about when you first wake up in the morning. What does your busy mind go to as it surges into consciousness?

What time is it?

Where do I have to be and when?

What's on my plate today?

Sometimes I go right to my first meeting or deadline in my mind, but then I course correct. That brief window of time after we wake up is critical to shaping our day. Our body is calibrating its stress and energy systems at that exact time. Our adrenal gland mounts a cortisol response into our blood when we wake up, even a little before that, as we unconsciously anticipate the day. Cortisol mobilizes as much glucose as our brain predicts it needs (thus its name, glucocorticoid). So, big day today? Better have a big cortisol spike! That's healthy—when we have huge demands and really need all that glucose in our blood! Around thirty minutes after we wake up, cortisol reaches its peak, and it can stick around a long time.

A big factor that shapes our waking cortisol is work stress. It may be hard to talk about overworking, but we need to: If we have chronically high levels of demand and responsibility at work, but few rewards like support and respect, then we end up with what researchers call "effort reward imbalance," a form of burnout from work. We tend to wake up with high cortisol, *and* we overshoot, having an excessive peak cortisol response that diminishes slowly.[26] This is especially true if we are mentally overcommitted to work—and our measure of overcommitment is not as good as it sounds. It's not dedication and purpose. Rather, it's being unable to stop thinking about work, disentangle, and relax. Overcommitment to work is also associated with having high cortisol before bedtime, our other critical period to guard.

Caregivers also suffer from this waking-up vigilance—because of their circumstances, they are particularly vulnerable to the habit of leaping forward in time: planning, anticipating, worrying. When we've studied healthy midlife parents, we've taken blood samples to look at the "youth" of their cells. At the same time, we look at their thought patterns when they wake and when they go to bed—those very important bookends of the day. We compare caregiving parents (those who have children with an autism diagnosis) with parents of neurotypical children. While all parents of young children are high stress, the caregiving parents have more accelerated cell aging and higher cortisol. But here's what's interesting.

Caregivers who wake up feeling positive—who feel joy, who describe feeling purpose in their role as caregiver, who find meaning in the difficult tasks they have to perform, who look forward to things in their day—have a better cellular aging profile, and they wake up with lower cortisol. They have a mindset that's oriented toward joy, and it shows in their bodies. They are more resilient. We've found that when people wake up feeling positivity about their day, or end their day with some positive emotions, they have higher levels of mitochondrial activity, along with higher levels of telomerase, the "antiaging enzyme."

Mitochondria are known as the "powerhouse" of the cell. They are our cell's batteries. They create energy called *adenosine triphosphate* (ATP), which fuels all of our essential cellular activity. Mitochondria are big, robust, and efficient when we're young; over time, as they age, they begin to create more oxidative stress. The older and weaker they get, the more oxidative stress leaks out, and the amount of energy they produce wanes. This is an important mind-body connection point: the average caregiving parent has lower-quality mitochondria, which can lead to less energy, less vitality. But caregiving parents with a positive emotion profile have high-quality mitochondria, just like noncaregiving parents.[27] Positive affect puts a kind of protective armor around them against stress, possibly even all the way down to the cellular level.

Your Mission: Start Full, End Full

The beginning of your day offers you a powerful opportunity to calibrate your nervous system. Like warm clay in your hands, your experience of your day is shaped as you shift your focus toward what you have, what you love, what you look forward to, what excites and interests you. It can be something as simple as thinking about how much you look forward to enjoying your first cup of coffee in the kitchen or loving up a furry companion.

The end of the day affects us powerfully as well. We want to go to bed without too much clutter and negative residue from the day on our minds. We need to wind down for restoration so we don't spend the night unconsciously stressing out. In today's practice, I'm going to ask you to try a simple ritual right before bed, designed to shift your mindset, tune your senses to your body and environment, and send cues to your body that it's okay to relax.

And for extra credit, I'll ask you to notice any little spark of joy you feel today. All the work we've done over the course of this book is so important, and these skills you've been working on are going to help you to be less triggered by stressors. But here's the wonderful thing about joy: when we increase it, we don't even need to reduce stress. Because the stress trigger just doesn't even go off—we have increased our stress threshold; it's harder to "see red."

The amazing thing about eudaimonic happiness is that it builds up your stress resilience. It gives you a deep well of reserve capacity—mental and emotional. When a stressor triggers a threat response for us, it's because we haven't managed to do the appropriate "mental triage"—we perceive something as threatening when, really, if we could just zoom out and get some perspective, we would see that sure, it's a challenge, but it's not a *threat*. We don't need to panic. We don't need to mount a huge threat stress response. Happiness and gratitude give us that reserve capacity, the charge to our battery. They give us solid ground to stand on. They give us the resources to zoom out, take a healthy perspective, see the challenge, stay flexible, and be resilient.

So today's practice is going to ask you to wake up, and to wind down, with gratitude, and to focus on what is meaningful to you. In the morning, it's about what you're looking forward to. In the evening, it's about reflecting on any moments of joy and satisfaction you experienced. Even throughout a difficult day, we can find these if we look carefully, and taking the time to focus on them may become the reason that the next day is even better, as we are able to meet it with greater resilience, openness, and joy.

TODAY'S PRACTICE

BLISS BOOKENDS

Go-Bag Skill: *Float on Joy*

Research shows that gratitude practices are one of the most powerful ways to shift our perspectives. Even for high school students, ten minutes a week of a gratitude exercise (writing letters to coaches, teachers, or friends, stating appreciation for something specific) led to increased feelings of connectedness and life satisfaction.[28] Gratitude counters hedonic adaptation, the well-documented effect in which after a pleasurable event, we quickly go back to a typical baseline level of emotion. We can fight hedonic adaptation by paying close attention to the positives in our lives, both big and small, and we know that the beginning and end of the day are the most effective times to do this. You might think of these as bliss bookends. Today's practice consists of two parts—a morning practice and an evening practice.

Morning Practice

As soon as you wake up, before getting out of bed, before picking up your phone, before you do anything, take five minutes to set a positive trajectory for your day today. You might sit up in bed to feel more alert. Let yourself gently awaken, with slow and easy breaths, to welcome the freshness of this new day. After taking three slow, mindful breaths, ask yourself:

What am I looking forward to today?

What am I grateful for?

The answer can be something as simple as *I'm looking forward to having a cup of strong coffee. I am grateful my partner did the food shopping so I have more personal time today. I'm happy to have a lunch date with someone I care about today.* Looking forward to aspects of your day—as opposed to spending your mental energy on planning for or dreading the tough stuff, and feeling only the sharp edges of the day—is a great way to cushion the day with "positive pillows." It's these little things each day that add up, buoy your spirit, and truly matter for your mental health.

If you wake up thinking about what you need to do—if that to-do list just adds up in your head—don't worry, that's okay. That's our natural, default mode of thinking. Remind yourself of something you care about in your day— something that matters to you. Feeling more daily purpose, reminding ourselves of why some task or obligation is meaningful, buffers us from stress and is even related to longevity.

Now, if you did pick up your phone, you didn't blow it! Check whatever you felt compelled to, put the phone down, and then take a few precious minutes to set your positive trajectory.

Evening Practice

When you climb into bed, take five minutes for joy practice. Your job here is to fill up your mind with the best thing that happened today.

What am I grateful for today?

Was there something that happened that went better than expected?

What made me smile or feel good today? Did I make someone smile today?

The tiniest things can be so powerful here. Even on a hard day, think back to the little moments: a hug from someone you care about, a kind interaction with a clerk, laughing with a colleague. The beauty of a flower. The love of a furry pet.

Finally, remember that the mind is recursive and ruminative. At the end of the day, let that work *for* you instead of against you. Think through the answers to the above questions as you fall asleep tonight—fill your mind with images of the moments that brought you joy today, that you'd like to savor a little bit longer. Let your body feel contentment and ease. This is how we "end full."

Bonus Practices

Make your bliss bookend a family affair! Try asking the evening questions above over dinner—have everyone take turns answering.

d a longer wind down before sleep for an even more powerful effect. The hour before you go to bed is a critical window. This is when you can start the descent toward good-quality sleep, which helps you to be less stressed the next day. Create a safe, secluded container by having quiet time: Make your to-do list for tomorrow, and turn off screens. Add a mind-body ritual if you like—yoga, stretching, breathing, or listening to soothing music. Now, feeling relaxed, this is the ideal time to do your gratitude practice. You may even fall asleep sooner, or have deeper sleep, the kind of sleep that gives your brain a good refresh.

For an even higher "positive balance" today, think of one small act of kindness you can do for someone else tomorrow. Social connections bring us joy. Having conversations or doing something kind for someone else—whether it's sharing a smile or a comment, making them feel seen, heard, less alone—these are the small things that actually create positive emotions in us and in others. And you can do this with anyone, not just people you already know. Acts of kindness toward strangers are small miracles that can have large effects. They are emotionally contagious.

Sometimes when I do something small for someone else, I find myself thinking about the small acts of kindness and grace in my own family's history that had significant ripple effects that the person performing the act never could have predicted. During the late 1800s, as a child, my great-grandmother was a refugee traveling alone without the correct papers. She was stopped by a ticket clerk as she tried to board a boat to safety. A bystander urged the clerk to let her board anyway, and after a moment of hesitation, the clerk nodded and waved her through. Perhaps that ticket clerk never thought about it again—or perhaps he did. I hope he got some joy out of that momentary act of compassion because without it, I would not exist. My late mother-in-law had a similar experience fleeing Germany as a child; if not for a clerk's empathy, seeing her expired passport but letting her onto a boat anyway, my son would not exist. I often think about these fleeting acts of kindness by those long-ago strangers with gratitude and wonder.

Perhaps you will find the opportunity to do something kind for someone else today.

Troubleshooting

If You Haven't Been Feeling Much Joy Lately and Aren't Sure Where to Look for It . . .

Ask yourself this question: What brings you joy? Joy from something you appreciate, or the small miracles you can find in a day. Don't ask yourself this just once—you won't get a full answer. Ask yourself eight times, answering as quickly as you can each time. So when in need of a solid boost, use this tactic. Don't hesitate. Just write down the first thing that comes to mind, then ask again. Doing this quickly allows you to bypass your inner censor. Surprise your mind; see what you find!

What brings you joy? _____

_____

What brings you joy? _____

_____

What brings you joy? _____

_____

What brings you joy? _____

_____

What brings you joy? _____

_____

What brings you joy? _____

_____

What brings you joy? _____

_____

What brings you joy? _____

_____

By answering rapidly over and over, you're less likely to prepare, judge, and think about a "right" response, allowing yourself to tap into what truly brings you joy. On retreats, we have people pair up and ask each other this question. When people are asked over and over, they don't know what will come out. So they discover! They find answers they weren't aware of. They often realize that they find joy in small things they did not previously recognize or value.

What happens after this exercise is truly a remarkable transformation. The energy level rises, and almost everyone in the room breaks out into smiles. People don't want to stop talking. We end the exercise by telling them, "Okay, write down what you discovered. Now you will shift your attention to these joyful moments even more."

On a Really Bad Day . . .

Try this: Was there any silver lining? Was someone kind? Was there something you learned?

If you're in the midst of a serious challenge, it might be really tough to see anything positive. Nevertheless, I encourage you to try to find one small positive thing from the day, or the week, and let yourself rest on that. Savor it. We also know that if you have serious depression, you might not be able to feel better right now. Depression is heavy. So rather than waiting until you're feeling better to do things that make you happy, do the reverse: schedule small activities that make you feel good, and do them regardless of your negative thoughts and feelings. This can help create positive affect and relieve depression.

These depths will not be forever. In tough times, I turn to some of my favorite quotes to remind me that hardships go hand in hand with joy. From Joanna Macy: "Falling apart is not such a bad thing. Indeed, it is as essential to evolutionary and psychological transformation as the cracking of outgrown shells." From Jane Hirshfield: "In order to gain anything, you must first lose everything."

Through adversity, we grow and gather more of the things that are meaningful: relationships, personal strength, wisdom. But this takes time, and for you, getting through the day is where the bar should be set. First and foremost, have self-compassion. Treat yourself with the utmost gentleness and kindness, as you would treat a best friend.

CONCLUSION

RENEWING YOUR PRESCRIPTION

WE STARTED THIS WEEK WITH A MISSION TO "PACK YOUR GO BAG" WITH the lightweight tools you need in order to be rested, ready, and resilient. Day by day, we built new "stress-resilience habits"— the more you practice these, the more cemented they'll become, replacing old modes of being that didn't serve you with ones that build ease and calm. My hope is that with the tools and tactics you've practiced this week, we can wipe out the single biggest source of our chronic stress: our worry about our uncertain future and all that we cannot control, regret and rumination about what didn't go as we'd hoped, and our attempt to battle these alone, in our heads.

This is a pivotal part of building stress resilience, because it turns out that we actually experience *two* distinct types of uncertainty. Since we cannot know the future, we have *irreducible uncertainty*, and we always will. Even in the most calm and stable of times, this type of uncertainty is always with us. It's the ever-present "unknowable" of what the next year will bring, the next week, tomorrow, the next hour. We all live with this—it's part of the human condition. But on top of that, we now also live with *volatile uncertainty*—rapid and unpredictable changes due to an uncertain physical and social world. Global challenges.

We are at an unusual point in history where we are experiencing new levels of volatile uncertainty and facing threats to our survival and to earth as we know it. Right now, things feel unstable. The world—both the physical, natural world and the social world—seems to be changing exponentially. Think about all that's thrown at us, every day: Extreme weather and an accelerating climate crisis. Political divisiveness and precariousness. Extremism and the wildfire spread of misinformation. A pandemic the likes of which none of us expected to see in our lifetimes, and the threat of more of the same.

It's overwhelming. It's humbling.

What I see in my research, and what I observe in people around me, is that we are getting lost in these existential crises, especially our youth. We are more threatened than ever by an uncertain future. Even the most resilient among us can be worn down by this, like a strong cliff eroding under rocky waves. We may at times lose meaning, direction, purpose; we are vulnerable to hopelessness and catastrophic thinking. And when we feel existentially threatened, it's hard to stand our ground and face the future with hope, resilience, flexibility, and a healthy challenge response.

But we still want to, and we can. Our children, our communities, and our planet need our best selves, our most creative thinking, and our collective action. And in an interesting twist, doing something toward repairing the world may be one of the most powerful ways to beat stress. So for our own well-being, and for the greater good, it's important that we renew our stress prescriptions, including "green prescriptions" to be with nature, and take excellent care of our mind and body, allowing deep restoration and joy. The future we are entering requires all our resources to survive, to thrive, together. And when we can come to a place of resilience and equanimity, we more fully enter an important state called the *plane of possibility*,[1] where we can break out of our personal thinking habits, understand our interconnectedness, and see new possibilities.

That's why this week has been all about building resilience: Bringing down your baseline levels of stress, both the stress you are aware of and the unconscious stress that lives in your body. Understanding how to access deep restoration. And ultimately creating healthier mind habits based on the best science we have available to us.

So let's recap the tools you now have available to you to do just that.

End-of-the-Week Inventory: What's in Your Go Bag?

You tried out seven new tactics over the course of this book, and I hope they have helped you to feel lighter, more flexible, more rested, more joyful, more able to *float*. I hope you are walking away from this stress-resilience training with a new approach to the stress in your life:

nexpected will happen, and that's okay. I can soften my expectations. I can lean back, relax, and let experiences come to me.

- I can let go of the things I can't control. I can drop the extra baggage.
- Stress can be exciting! I can feel motivated and energized by challenges.
- I can relax into acute stress and metabolize it. My body loves a good stress response.
- I can let nature do the work of recalibrating my nervous system. I am part of nature.
- I deserve rest. I will no longer starve myself of relaxation, sleep, and deep rest.
- Joy shrinks stress. The more I fill my cup with joy, the less I can taste the bitterness of stress and struggle.

We said at the beginning of this book that stress is the water we swim in, but that we could learn strategies to help us float, to ride the waves of stress instead of getting swamped by them. Using the skills you've learned this week, you can. I like to think of it this way: I'm guiding my boat down a unfamiliar river. I have choices throughout my day and my life—I can choose this fork or that one as the water branches off, but the current runs only one way. I don't control the flow of the water, and while I can maneuver a bit as conditions allow, I can't paddle upstream— I'll only wear myself out. Guiding myself skillfully down this river means embracing the unexpected, taking in experiences as they arise, tackling the rocks and rapids with a challenge mindset, controlling what I can, and staying afloat through the rest. We can even pause, let the water swirl gently around us. When we lean back and shift toward green and blue mind states, feel ease and contentment, we are sending strong messages to our cells that it is time to rest and restore.

It's too easy to feel overwhelmed, to spend our time in red and yellow mind states. When we realize that things are always changing, that we don't control the future, that we can only do our best, we can be open to what emerges, to the joy that is hidden in every day.

Here, at a glance, is your stress prescription. You can see the names of the practices for each strategy, to trigger your memory. Consider putting this on your refrigerator!

DAY 1	DAY 2	DAY 3	DAY 4	DAY 5	DAY 6	DAY 7
Embrace Uncertainty	Let Go of What You Can't Control	Find Excitement in Challenges	Metabolize Body Stress	Immerse Yourself in Nature	Experience Deep Rest	Create Bliss Bookends
Releasing Embodied Stress	Stress Inventory	Stress Shield	Hormetic Stress	Sensory Absorption	Breathe for Restoration	Start and End Full of Joy
• Identifying embodied stress • Noting expectations and worries • Breathing into it, releasing	• Simplifying: What can I delete? • Adding: What matters most? • Putting down: What can I accept?	• Positive stress mindset • Reaffirm your values • Recall your resources and reframe toward resilience	• HIIT or brisk walking • Cold showers • Hot sauna • Relaxing into discomfort	• Wild nature • Urban nature • Home sanctuary	• Breathe (long, slow, deep) for wellness • 4-6-8 breathing for resetting • Vagal breathing for relaxation	• Noticing joy • Living daily purpose • Expressing gratitude • Kindness inward and outward

The preceding "prescription" for stress resilience is your skill set for our unknown future. To tackle the challenges ahead, we will need a calm, flexible mindset. And finally, we need hope.

"Active Hope" Will Help You Float

Extreme uncertainty leads to the destruction of our most important human source of resilience: radical hope in humankind and in our future. And hope isn't just a feeling. It's about *action*. Joanna Macy calls it "active hope," and in her description, she includes both *self-care* and *other care*. In short, take care of yourself, make time to restore, *and* find a way to give back: make change, move the needle on something that matters to you—however small you feel it is. It will help you; it will add up; it will help us all.

Macy has a vow each day to renew her purpose and align her actions. The Dalai Lama also has a daily vow that helps him live a purposeful, committed life. In my dialogue with him, I asked how we can have hope in the face of the overwhelming existential problems we currently confront. He replied that recognizing and focusing on whatever bit of progress we've already made can give us some space to feel courage and confidence, necessary companions to hope. The alternative—fixating attention on our problems—obscures clear thinking. He shared his own daily strategy: he recites vows from the Indian master Shantideva each morning. "What gives me courage and confidence is the continual renewal of warmheartedness. . . . I find reflecting on these verses to be very helpful. What we need is a way to

ew our positive intention." He points to a particu-
l those happy in the world are so because of their de-
ppiness of others[2]—and explains, "If we focus too
much on ourselves, we'll not be happy even in this life, whereas
to concern ourselves with the well-being of others is the gate-
way to great joy."[3]

These are hard times; a daily hope vow is a wise addition to our
stress practices, and to starting every day full. You could make
up a vow if that helps you, or you might already have one from
your spiritual or religious tradition. I like to try new ones, and
love to learn what others use. Here is one of my favorites to start
the day, an excerpt from a prayer written by Pádraig Ó Tuama:[4]

> *We begin our day alone, honoring this life with all its
> potentials and possibilities.*
>
> *We begin our day with hope, knowing the day can hold love,
> kindness, forgiveness, and justice.*
>
> *May we make room for the unexpected. May we find wisdom
> and life in the unexpected.*

Active hope is stronger than abstract hope. It's not fragile.
It's durable. It's hope infused with caring action. It can't be easily lost. It can't be eroded or washed away by uncertainty and
threat. And it's a highly contagious emotion because it inspires
others to do the same. It spreads social change. And it's one of

the most powerful things you can do to find relief from stress, pain, sorrow, anxiety, and anger. That's why, here at the end of our week together, we are adding one more tool for stress resilience: a sense of purpose.

Your go bag is light. Purpose will lighten it even further. Think of it as helium that lightens your step and buoys you along.

Keep an Eye on Your "North Star"

We talked earlier about deleting stressors when we can—especially those that we've put on ourselves and believe we "must" do. Social obligations can fit into this category, or other kinds of "keeping-up" activities in which we add responsibilities and stress at work or in our communities because we feel pressure. We're going to stick with that. And hopefully shedding some of that stress will leave us with a little room, a little breathing space, to consider: *What's truly important to me? What do I want to spend my life energy on? What is my North Star?*

People often tell me they are "in survival mode." They feel like their personal life is a mess and they can't take on anything else. But then there's a counterintuitive truth at the center of everything: doing something outside of ourselves gives us active hope and purpose. It actually lifts our spirit and reduces stress.

Perhaps what we need most of all to carry stress well is purpose.

You don't need to have everything figured out to access this.

We often operate within a mindset of *I'm going to get my life in order*, then *I'm going to think about doing something I've been wanting to do that's for the greater good*. But you don't have to have mastered your daily drama. It's not going to go away.

I will always remember the morning, in the late summer of 2020, when those of us on the West Coast woke up on Mars. The sky was brick red. The air was toxic. The heavy smoke from devastating wildfires had settled high above San Francisco and blocked the sun. Our mailman needed to use a headlamp to deliver the mail at 10:00 a.m.

My distress over these growing climate problems was increasing. I was thinking about it more, wanting to talk about it more. But I was "full."

The demands of my job as a professor, teaching and running the lab, along with my roles at home and as a caretaker, were relentless as they always had been. But at a certain point, I realized I couldn't live like that any longer. I decided to cross over, to go from being a climate worrier to a climate warrior, in whatever way I could be effective.

It's been challenging, because the climate crisis feels overwhelming. Our emotions might swing back and forth, from despair and sadness to hope and joy—like a metronome—so much that we feel whiplash. There are so many changes we need, large and small, and it's often hard to feel like you're having an effect. I've had ideas for projects but felt stymied, like they wouldn't be enough. I developed more robust hope in part by learning about the theory of quantum social change, which helps us see that changing things locally—the tangible factors within our own sphere of influence—will actually have contagious and rippling impacts.[5] In this way, together we can change aspects of our culture. Even if we cannot see our impact, and may never in our lifetime, what we do as individuals matters.

I am beginning a project to move people from climate distress to climate action. This is a special class to provide information and skills that we hope will inspire people to make change without feeling hopeless or overwhelmed. We are using the principles we've been talking about—being able to hold joy amid sadness and anger, feeling empowered by purpose and working with others—and really putting the quantum social change into action. I don't know how it will turn out. But I do know the best way to reduce climate despair is through some type of climate-related action.

One thing that's clear from the science: having purpose in your life is stress buffering. When I work on climate issues, I feel a buzz of positive energy, that I am living fully, the way I would if I knew my time on earth were ending soon. This certainty—that I'm doing something that matters to me—helps me better handle all the other uncertainties of life.

You might already be working on what gives you strong purpose. If not, think about the things you've been *wanting* to do. Even adding an hour a week of a passion project can be meaningful.

Doing something more right now, adding to your busy day, might not sound feasible if you're struggling to keep your head above water. There are other ways to get the stress-buffering effects of purpose than adding something new. Sometimes we just need to realize the purpose that is already there, the things we already do that are meaningful to others. Take a moment now to consider the things you are already doing that give you purpose. We often simply don't see the impact we're having.

You Already Make a Difference

We all have influence. You are contributing in unquantified ways to the world around you, ways that might have repercussions and influence beyond your knowledge—and beyond your life.

My father, David, is a retired biology professor. After his retirement party, he received a letter from a student he'd taught twenty years earlier. My father was delighted to hear from him. But the best surprise was about his hidden impact.

This student had been struggling with a bad case of impostor syndrome. He came from a small town, and at Stanford he felt like a little fish in a big sea—like he didn't really belong. He believed Stanford had made a mistake letting him in. He earned Bs and Cs and didn't think of himself as a top student among stars. One summer, he came to my father's lab to do marine biology research, and excelled at it. When my father saw his transcript of grades, he said, "Well, that isn't right. I know you, and I know you can do better than that."

This student mulled over these comments and decided they could be true. He went on to get excellent grades and eventually become a world-class surgeon. He wrote because he wanted my father to know that a single conversation showing confidence in him had changed his life trajectory. For my father, the whole incident represented just a fleeting interaction—the kind of thing he did with students all the time. But it had made an enormous impact. And in turn, this beautiful letter has had its own unknown impact. My father cherishes this letter in his retirement, a decade later.

Everyone can ask themselves: *What am I really doing, beyond what I can see?*

There are so many unnamed and unknown positive influences. You don't have to have any particular type of job in order to have a big impact. Someone doing art as a hobby can think about the message they want to communicate to the world. Someone staying home to raise their children can think about the love and support they are offering this little person, helping them to become another human in the world doing good, in their own small but important way. What is the long-term impact of what *you* are doing? You can't fully know—and that's actually a beautiful thing.

We talked about the fear that can come from uncertainty. But there's also *possibility*. We don't know what impact we might have, what small acts of kindness and generosity will make a huge difference for someone, which efforts we make for the common good will cause ripple effects. It could be profound. We don't know how we might transform our society together, but it is a possibility.

Yes, uncertainty can be stressful—but it also means the door is open to life's surprises. It means the future will bring challenges but also beauty, awe, gratitude, and joy. A resilient mind opens up a world of possibility. When you catch yourself tightening up, try the opposite: Release the tension. Release the control you never really had. Smile at uncertainty. Uncertainty also means *freedom*.

Anything can happen.

Your life is full of possibility.

Take that weightless go bag, filled with the tools you need to meet each challenge, and go out and live it.

ACKNOWLEDGMENTS

I am grateful to many colleagues and friends who helped me write this book, which despite its small size required lots of support! First of all, thanks to Idea Architects, Rachel Neumann and Doug Abrams, for their optimism that stress could be hacked in seven days, for their trust in me and for their stewardship of the book, and especially to Alyssa Knickerbocker for her fantastic writing support and contagious joy. Deep gratitude to Amy Sun of Penguin Life, for her careful curation and editing with surgical precision.

A deep thanks to my many colleagues who have been part of this stress prescription in some way, including making sure study details get transmuted into accurate and useful messages, especially Amit Bernstein, George Bonanno, Alexandra Crosswell, Alia Crum, David Creswell, Martica Hall, Dacher Keltner, Paul Lehrer, Robert Lustig, Sonja Lyubomirsky, Ashley Mason, Patrick McKeown, Wallace Nichols, Martin Picard, Eli Puterman, Charles Raison, Michael Sapiro, Cliff Saron, Shauna Shapiro, Emiliana Simon Thomas, Victor Strecher, Julian Thayer, Cassandra Vieten, and Eric Zimmerman.

A special thanks to my close collaborators in our center at UCSF, who help make research and challenging studies so much fun—Aric Prather and Wendy Mendes and our wonderful team at the Aging, Metabolism and Emotion Center. Thanks to Elizabeth Blackburn and Jue Lin, for the decades-long friendship and dialogue about resilience of our telomeres, from molecules to mind. Thank you to my many colleagues in our Department of Psychiatry and Behavioral Sciences, making the pandemic period one of connection and support despite heavy burden and Zoom fatigue. Thank you to Lisa Pritzker, Sako Fisher, Joon Yun, and Lynne and Victor Brick, for special support. Thank you to my lifelong mentors Nancy Adler, Kelly Brownell, Philip Zimbardo, and the late Albert Bandura.

Thank you to the many friends and devoted wisdom teachers who have directly or indirectly helped with my own stress resilience over many years—James Baraz, Peter and Alison Baumann, Mark Coleman, Richard Davidson, Eve Ekman, Lama Willa Miller, Lama Tsultrim Allione, Joanie Kriens, Jack Kornfield, Trudy Goodman, Roshi Joan Halifax, Stephan Rechtschaffen, Annette Knopp, Esther Perel, Jack Saul, Dan Siegel, Tempel Smith, Bhikkhu Anālayo, Caroline Welch, Rick and Jan Hanson, Jon Kabat Zinn, Will and Teresa Kabat-Zinn, Darrah Westrup, and colleagues from the NeuroDharma group. A deep bow to my dear friend Susan Bauer-Wu and wonderful colleagues at the Mind & Life Institute and its Steering Council, for cocreating precious forums where magical alchemy of science and contemplative wisdom takes place. These have shaped my own mind and life.

It was a gift to have a sophisticated group of readers improve an early version, especially with their own experiences of the practices, including Cathy Caplener, Ron Chiarello, Elisabeth Doehring, Andrew Dreitcer, Mark Godley, Jeannette Ickovics, Amy Lauer, Robert Lustig, Dan Meer, Peter Prontzos, Jamey Schmidt, Ally and Lilia Shirman, Tracy Turner, David Vogel, Julia Wallace, and especially Lynn Kutler.

Thank you to my wonderful extended family, and the nucleus—David and Lois Epel, sisters Sharon Epel and Andrea Lieberstein, Danny Glaser, and of course my beloved, Jack Glaser. And . . . lastly, my gratitude to you, the reader, for trusting me to advise you, for your open mind to try something new from this set of ideas. May it bring more ease to your one precious life.

FURTHER READING AND RESOURCES

If you'd like to go further with any of the skills we practiced here, I've compiled some of my favorite books and web-based resources. These are also available online at www.elissaepel.com so you can access the links easily.

TO CONTINUE WORKING ON DAY 1 SKILLS: UNCERTAINTY STRESS

Standing at the Edge: Finding Freedom Where Fear and Courage Meet, by Joan Halifax and Rebecca Solnit. New York: Flatiron Books, 2018. (Adversity and edge states can lead us to our best qualities).

In Love with the World: A Monk's Journey through the Bardos of Living and Dying, 1st ed., by Yongey Mingyur Rinpoche and Helen Tworkov. New York: Random House, 2019. (Rinpoche describes the mind states the allow us to live with joy while under great uncertainty stress.)

Any meditation app, such as *10% Happier*, *HeadSpace*, the free *Insight Timer*, or *Healthy Minds* program app: https://hminnovations.org/meditation-app. To hear a top Buddhist teacher, Bikkhu Analayo provides mindfulness of breathing meditations at: https://www.buddhistinquiry.org/resources/offerings-analayo/breathing-audio/.

TO CONTINUE WORKING ON DAY 2 SKILLS:
LETTING GO OF CONTROL

The Serenity Prayer (adapted serenity prayer from Alcoholics Anonymous recovery programs): "May I have the serenity to accept the things I cannot change, courage to change the things I can, and the wisdom to know the difference."

Feeding Your Demons: Ancient Wisdom for Resolving Inner Conflict, 1st ed., by Lama Tsultrim Allione. New York: Little, Brown Spark, 2008. (This technique uses visualization to give shape and color to our "demons"—our negative emotional responses to a relationship or situation—and transforms them into a strength.)

The Burnout Challenge: Managing People's Relationships with Their Jobs, by Christina Maslach and Michael Leiter. Cambridge, MA: Harvard University Press, 2022.

The Dialectical Behavior Therapy Skills Workbook: Practical DBT Exercises for Learning Mindfulness, Interpersonal Effectiveness, Emotion Regulation, and Distress Tolerance, 2nd ed., by Matthew McKay, PhD, Jeffrey C. Wood, PsyD, and Jeffrey Brantley, MD. Oakland, CA: New Harbinger, 2019.

TO CONTINUE WORKING ON DAY 3 SKILLS:
POSITIVE STRESS MIND STATES TO COMBAT DAILY STRESS, ANXIETY, AND DEPRESSION

Breaking the Age Code: How Your Beliefs about Aging Determine How Long and Well You Live, by Becca Levy. New York: William Morrow, 2022.

Resilient: How to Grow an Unshakable Core of Calm, Strength, and Happiness, by Rick Hanson and Forrest Hanson. New York: Harmony, 2022. https://www.rickhanson.net/resilient/.

The Upside of Stress: Why Stress Is Good for You, and How to Get Good at It, by Kelly McGonigal. New York: Avery, 2016.

For employers: Meru Health, https://www.meruhealth.com/. This is a self-help app platform for depression and anxiety, providing evidence-based therapy, biofeedback of heart rate variability, and sessions with therapists trained in mindfulness-based cognitive therapy. (Note my conflict of interest; I am on their advisory board.)

TO CONTINUE WORKING ON DAY 4 SKILLS: HORMETIC STRESS

The Wim Hof Method: Activate Your Full Human Potential, by Wim Hof, foreword by Elissa Epel. Louisville, CO: Sounds True, 2020.

The Better Brain: Overcome Anxiety, Combat Depression, and Reduce ADHD and Stress with Nutrition by Bonnie Kaplan and Julia Rucklidge. Boston: Houghton Mifflin Harcourt, 2021. (This book describes how diet patterns and micronutrients improve mental health. In addition, certain plant chemicals work partly through hormetic stress processes).

Which types of exercise help with which types of mental health issues? Explore this interactive website for a comprehensive report: https://www.johnwbrick foundation.org/move-your-mental-health-report/.

It is easy to find high intensity interval training videos on the internet: Peloton has classes online, as well as Lanebreak, a HIIT workout disguised as a game.

TO CONTINUE WORKING ON DAY 5 SKILLS: RECALIBRATING YOUR NERVOUS SYSTEM WITH NATURE

Blue Mind: The Surprising Science That Shows How Being Near, in, on, or Under Water Can Make You Happier, Healthier, More Connected, and Better at What You Do, by Wallace J. Nichols. New York: Little, Brown and Company, 2015.

"The Mind, the Human-Earth Connection and the Climate Crisis Online Course" from the Mind and Life Summer Research Institute, a free seminar available here: https://www.mindandlife.org/climate-online-course/. (With my colleagues, we have featured top international speakers in a contemplative course with rich information on developing climate resilience and healing our relationship with nature.)

For nature retreats, search online or create your own! I recommend Mark Coleman's guided nature retreats and nature mindfulness teacher training: https://markcoleman.org/.

TO CONTINUE WORKING ON DAY 6 SKILLS: EXPERIENCING DEEP REST

The Wakeful Body: Somatic Mindfulness as a Path to Freedom, by Willa Baker and Tsoknyi Rinpoche. Boulder, CO: Shambhala, 2021. (This beautifully written book describes subtle body energy, a way to tune in to unconscious stress and find ease).

The Breathing Cure: Develop New Habits for a Healthier, Happier, and Longer Life, by Patrick McKeown and Laird Hamilton. New York: Humanix Books, 2021. (This comprehensive book offers tailored breathing exercises for many conditions).

Residential retreat centers for meditation or yoga: When possible, it's wonderful to pack light and go inward for a deep reset by having at least a few days at a spiritual, meditation, or yoga retreat center that is not also for commercial tourism. I recommend three meditation retreat centers that I know well, below. Most states have options that can be found on the web. This site lists spiritual retreats around the world: https://www.spiritualtravels.info /spiritual-sites-around-the-world/.

• Insight Meditation Society, Barre, MA: https://www.dharma.org/.
• Spirit Rock Meditation Center, Woodacre, CA: https://www.spiritrock.org/.
• Wonderwell Mountain Refuge, New Hampshire: https://naturaldharma.org/.

Try these free guided meditations for well-being and for sleep: https://www .irest.org/try-irest-now.

Consider using a wearable biosensor to help you know what works best for you, and how your nervous system responds during practices and during sleep. My favorite is the Oura ring (oura.com). Try heart rate variability feedback such as with the HeartMath product found here: https://store.heartmath.org/.

TO CONTINUE WORKING ON DAY 7 SKILLS: JOY AND "POSITIVE PILLOWS"

Awakening Joy: 10 Steps to Happiness, by James Baraz, Shoshana Alexander, Ram Dass, Jack Kornfield. New York: Ballantine Books, 2012.

Greater Good in Action (GGIA): This website, https://ggia.berkeley.edu/, is an extensive catalog of activities, exercises, and practices for strengthening skills that promote emotional well-being like awe, gratitude, and compassion. These are drawn from published scientific research, and studies of engagement and impact are directed by my colleagues Dacher Keltner and Emiliana Simon Thomas.

The Big Joy Project (research): This website and mobile app, at https://ggia .berkeley.edu/bigjoy, is a one-week experience I have created in collaboration with my research colleagues Peggy Callahan and Jolene Smith of the Mission Joy campaign, and UCB's Greater Good Science Center, to promote inner joy and well-being. This is also a citizen science project to discover more about what works for whom, across different regions and countries. Please share this if you like it!

Mission: Joy—Finding Happiness in Troubled Times, a documentary about joy amid adversity, and the friendship between His Holiness the Dalai Lama and Archbishop Desmond Tutu. https://missionjoy.org/.

Tank's Good News: Counter the negative daily news! I cannot help but laugh or smile reading the daily post on Instagram (@tanksgoodnews). Or you can get the newsletter at https://tanksgoodnews.com.

TO KEEP "RENEWING YOUR PRESCRIPTION" (CONCLUSION):

You Matter More Than You Think: Quantum Social Change for a Thriving World, by Karen O'Brien, and Christina Bethell, Oslo, Norway: cChange, 2021.

Humanity Rising is a global broadcast that started with the pandemic, convened by Ubiquity University, with viewers in 130 countries. It provides dialogue by thought leaders addressing global issues and how to build resilience and renewal to ensure the human future. You might feel inspired and more connected globally. https://humanityrising.solutions/.

One Earth Sangha: https://oneearthsangha.org/., offers classes and webinars on how to approach the climate crisis from both an engaged active and a contemplative perspective.

Regeneration.org: Get started here on climate change action.

Purpose: Living for What Matters Most, a free course on Coursera by Professor Victor Strecher.

NOTES

INTRODUCTION

1. Jue Lin and Elissa Epel, "Stress and Telomere Shortening: Insights from Cellular Mechanisms," *Ageing Research Reviews 73* (January 2022): 101507, https://doi.org/10.1016/j.arr.2021.101507.
2. David M. Almeida, Susan T. Charles, Jacqueline Mogle, Johanna Drewelies, Carolyn M. Aldwin, Avron Spiro III, and Denis Gerstorf, "Charting Adult Development through (Historically Changing) Daily Stress Processes," *American Psychologist* 75, no. 4 (May–June 2020): 511–24, https://doi.org/10.1037/amp0000597.
3. Achim Peters, Bruce S. McEwen, and Karl Friston, "Uncertainty and Stress: Why It Causes Diseases and How It Is Mastered by the Brain," *Progress in Neurobiology* 156 (September 2017): 164–88, https://doi.org/10.1016/j.pneurobio.2017.05.004.
4. Alexandra Crosswell, Stefanie Mayer, Lauren Whitehurst, Sheyda Zebarjadian, Martin Picard, and Elissa Epel, "Deep Rest: An Integrative Model of How Contemplative Practices Enhance the Body's Restorative Capacity" (under review).
5. Jos F. Brosschot, Bart Verkuil, and Julian F. Thayer, "Generalized Unsafety Theory of Stress: Unsafe Environments and Conditions, and the Default Stress Response," in "Stress and Health," ed. Mark Cropley, Birgitta Gatersleben, and Stefan Sütterlin, special issue, *International*

Journal of Environmental Research and Public Health 15, no. 3 (March 7, 2018): 464, https://doi.org/10.3390/ijerph15030464.

6. His Holiness the Dalai Lama, "Mind and Life Conversation: Embracing Hope, Courage, and Compassion in Times of Crisis," interview by Elissa Epel and Michelle Shiota, moderated by John Dunne, Mind and Life Institute, December 8, 2021, 1:18:01, www.mindandlife.org/event/embracing-hope-courage-and-compassion/.

DAY 1: THINGS WILL GO WRONG . . . AND THAT'S ALL RIGHT

1. Natalia Bobba-Alves et al. "Chronic Glucocorticoid Stress Reveals Increased Energy Expenditure and Accelerated Aging as Cellular Features of Allostatic Load," *BioRxiv* (2022), https://doi.org/10.1101/2022.02.22.481548.

2. Archy O. de Berker, Robb B. Rutledge, Christoph Mathys, Louise Marshall, Gemma F. Cross, Raymond J. Dolan, and Sven Bestmann, "Computations of Uncertainty Mediate Acute Stress Responses in Humans," *Nature Communications* 7 (March 29, 2016): 10996, https://doi.org/10.1038/ncomms10996.

3. Dilek Celik, Emre H. Alpay, Betul Celebi, and Aras Turkali, "Intolerance of Uncertainty, Rumination, Post-Traumatic Stress Symptoms and Aggression during COVID-19: A Serial Mediation Model," *European Journal of Psychotraumatology* 12, no. 1 (August 13, 2021): 1953790, https://doi.org/10.1080/20008198.2021.1953790.

4. Yuanyuan Gu, Simeng Gu, Yi Lei, and Hong Li, "From Uncertainty to Anxiety: How Uncertainty Fuels Anxiety in a Process Mediated by Intolerance of Uncertainty," in "Stress Induced Neuroplasticity and Mental Disorders 2020," ed. Fang Pan, Lee Shapiro, and Jason H. Huang, special issue, *Neural Plasticity* 2020 (October 1, 2020): 8866386, https://doi.org/10.1155/2020/8866386

5. Jessica C. Jimenez, Katy Su, Alexander R. Goldberg, Victor M. Luna, Jeremy S. Biane, Gokhan Ordek, Pengcheng Zhou et al., "Anxiety Cells in a Hippocampal-Hypothalamic Circuit," *Neuron* 97, no. 3 (February 7, 2018): 670–83.e6, https://doi.org/10.1016/j.neuron.2018.01.016..

6. Marc-Lluís Vives and Oriel FeldmanHall, "Tolerance to Ambiguous Uncertainty Predicts Prosocial Behavior," *Nature Communications* 9 (June 12, 2018): 2156, https://doi.org/10.1038/s41467-018-04631-9.

7. Jeroen M. van Baar, David J. Halpern, and Oriel FeldmanHall, "Intolerance of Uncertainty Modulates Brain-to-Brain Synchrony during Politically Polarized Perception, *Proceedings of the National Academy of Sciences* 118, no. 20 (May 13, 2021): e2022491118, https://doi.org/10.1073/pnas.2022491118.

8. Andreas B. Neubauer, Joshua M. Smyth, and Martin J. Sliwinski, "When

You See It Coming: Stressor Anticipation Modulates Stress Effects on Negative Affect," *Emotion* 18, no. 3 (April 2018): 342–54, https://doi.org/10.1037/emo0000381.

9. Kirstin Aschbacher, Aoife O'Donovan, Owen M. Wolkowitz, Firdaus S. Dhabhar, Yali Su, and Elissa Epel, "Good Stress, Bad Stress and Oxidative Stress: Insights from Anticipatory Cortisol Reactivity," *Psychoneuroendocrinology* 38, no. 9 (September 2013): 1698–708, https://doi.org/10.1016/j.psyneuen.2013.02.004.

10. Roxane Cohen Silver, E. Alison Holman, and Dana Rose Garfin. "Coping with Cascading Collective Traumas in the United States," *Nature Human Behavior* 5, no. 1 (January 2021): 4–6, https://doi.org/10.1038/s41562-020-00981-x.

11. Roxane Cohen Silver, E. Alison Holman, Judith Pizarro Andersen, Michael Poulin, Daniel N. McIntosh, and Virginia Gil-Rivas, "Mental- and Physical-Health Effects of Acute Exposure to Media Images of the September 11, 2001, Attacks and the Iraq War," *Psychological Science* 24, no. 9 (September 2013): 1623–34, https://doi.org/10.1177/0956797612460406.

DAY 2: CONTROL WHAT YOU CAN . . . AND PUT DOWN THE REST

1. Stephanie A. Robinson and Margie E. Lachman, "Perceived Control and Aging: A Mini-Review and Directions for Future Research," *Gerontology* 63, no. 5 (August 2017): 435–42, https://doi.org/10.1159/000468540.

2. Shevaun D. Neupert, David M. Almeida, and Susan Turk Charles, "Age Differences in Reactivity to Daily Stressors: The Role of Personal Control," *Journals of Gerontology: Series B* 62, no. 4 (July 2007): P216–25, https://doi.org/10.1093/geronb/62.4.p216.

3. Laura L. Carstensen, Yochai Z. Shavit, and Jessica T. Barnes, "Age Advantages in Emotional Experience Persist Even under Threat from the COVID-19 Pandemic," *Psychological Science* 31, no. 11 (November 2020): 1374–1385, https://doi.org/10.1177/0956797620967261.

4. Carol A. Shively and Stephen M. Day, "Social Inequalities in Health in Nonhuman Primates," *Neurobiology of Stress* 1 (January 2015): 156–63, https://doi.org/10.1016/j.ynstr.2014.11.005.

5. Jay R. Kaplan, Haiying Chen, and Stephen B. Manuck, "The Relationship between Social Status and Atherosclerosis in Male and Female Monkeys as Revealed by Meta-analysis," in "Special Issue on Nonhuman Primate Models of Women's Health," ed. Carol A. Shively and Thomas B. Clarkson, *American Journal of Primatology* 71, no. 9 (September 2009): 732–41, https://doi.org/10.1002/ajp.20707.

6. Janice K. Kiecolt-Glaser, Phillip T. Marucha, W. B. Malarkey, Ana M. Mercado, and Ronald Glaser, "Slowing of Wound Healing by Psychological Stress," *The Lancet* 346, no. 8984 (November 4, 1995): 1194–96, https://doi.org/10.1016/S0140-6736(95)92899-5.

7. Saher Hoda Kamil and Dawn I. Velligan, "Caregivers of Individuals with Schizophrenia: Who Are They and What Are Their Challenges?," *Current Opinion in Psychiatry* 43, no. 3 (May 2019): 157–63, https://doi.org/10.1097/YCO.0000000000000492.

8. Anna Sjörs Dahlman, Ingibjörg H.Jonsdottir, and Caroline Hansson, "The Hypothalamo-pituitary-adrenal Axis and the Autonomic Nervous System in Burnout," in "The Human Hypothalamus: Neuropsychiatric Disorders," ed. Dick F. Swaab, Ruud M. Buijs, Felix Kreier, Paul J. Lucassen, and Ahmad Salehi, *Handbook of Clinical Neurology* 182 (2021): 83–94, https://doi.org/10.1016/B978-0-12-819973-2.00006-X.

9. Christina Maslach and Michael P. Leiter, *The Burnout Challenge: Managing People's Relationships with Their Jobs* (Cambridge, MA: Harvard University Press, 2022).

10. Annie Dillard, *The Writing Life* (New York: HarperCollins, 1989)

11. Hsiao-Wen Liao and Laura L. Carstensen, "Future Time Perspective: Time Horizons and Beyond," in "Future Time Perspectives," special issue, *GeroPsych* 31, no. 3 (September 2018): 163–67, https://doi.org/10.1024/1662-9647/a000194.

12. Marsha M. Linehan, *DBT Skills Training Mannual*, 2nd ed. (New York: Guilford Publications, 2015). DBT, or Dialectical Behavioral Therapy, includes the practices of Radical Acceptance.

13. Alexandra D. Crosswell, Michael Coccia, and Elissa S. Epel, "Mind Wandering and Stress: When You Don't Like the Present Moment," *Emotion* 20, no. 3 (April 2020): 403–12, https://doi.org/10.1037/emo0000548.

14. Elissa S. Epel, Eli Puterman, Jue Lin, Elizabeth Blackburn, Alanie Lazaro, and Wendy Berry Mendes, "Wandering Minds and Aging Cells," *Clinical Psychological Science* 1, no. 1 (January 2013): 75–83, https://doi.org/10.1177/2167702612460234.

15. Steven Hayes and Spencer Smith, *Get out of Your Mind and into Your Life: The New Acceptance and Commitment Therapy* (Oakland, CA: New Harbinger Publications, 2015).

16. Emily K. Lindsay, ShinzenYoung, Joshua M. Smyth, Kirk Warren Brown, and J. David Creswell, "Acceptance Lowers Stress Reactivity: Dismantling Mindfulness Training in a Randomized Controlled Trial," *Psychoneuroendocrinology* 87 (January 2018): 63–73, https://doi.org/10.1016/j.psyneuen.2017.09.015.

17. Emily K. Lindsay, Brian Chin, Carol M. Greco, Shinzen Young, Kirk W. Brown, Aidan G. C. Wright, Joshua M. Smyth, Deanna Burkett, and J. David Creswell, "How Mindfulness Training Promotes Positive Emotions: Dismantling Acceptance Skills Training in Two Randomized Controlled Trials," *Journal of Personality and Social Psychology* 115, no. 6 (December 2018): 944–73, https://doi.org/10.1037/pspa0000134.

18. Nora Görg, Kathlen Priebe, Jan R. Böhnke, Regina Steil, Anne S. Dyer, and Nikolaus Kleindienst, "Trauma-Related Emotions and Radical Acceptance in Dialectical Behavior Therapy for Posttraumatic Stress Disorder after Childhood Sexual Abuse," *Borderline Personality Disorder and Emotion Dysregulation* 4 (July 13, 2017): 15, https://doi.org/10.1186/s40479-017-0065-5; and Jenny Thorsell Cederberg, Martin Cernvall, JoAnne Dahl, Louise von Essen, and Gustaf Ljungman, "Acceptance as a Mediator for Change in Acceptance and Commitment Therapy for Persons with Chronic Pain?," *International Journal of Behavioral Medicine* 23, no. 1 (February 2016): 21–29, https://doi.org/10.1007/s12529-015-9494-y.

DAY 3: BE THE LION

1. Elissa S. Epel, Alexandra D. Crosswell, Stefanie E. Mayer, Aric A. Prather, George M. Slavich, Eli Puterman, and Wendy Berry Mendes, "More Than a Feeling: A Unified View of Stress Measurement for Population Science," *Frontiers in Neuroendocrinology* 49 (April 2018): 146–69, https://doi.org/10.1016/j.yfrne.2018.03.001.

2. Stefanie E. Mayer, Agus Surachman, Aric A. Prather, Eli Puterman, Kevin L. Delucchi, Michael R. Irwin, Andrea Danese, David M. Almeida, and Elissa S. Epel, "The Long Shadow of Childhood Trauma for Depression in Midlife: Examining Daily Psychological Stress Processes as a Persistent Risk Pathway," *Psychological Medicine* (March 26, 2021): 1–10, https://doi.org/10.1017/S0033291721000921.

3. Joanna Guan, Elaz Ahmadi, Bresh Merino, Lindsay Fox, K. Miller, J. Kim, and Stefanie Mayer. "Developing Stress Resilience in Everyday Life—Examining Stress Appraisal Effects of an Ecological Mindfulness Intervention Developed for Midlife Women with a History of Early Life Adversity." (Poster presentation online at the 7th International Symposium on Resilience Research, International Resilience Alliance Intresa, September 2021).

4. Elissa Epel, Jennifer Daubenmier, Judith Tedlie Moskowitz, Susan Folkman, and Elizabeth Blackburn, "Can Meditation Slow Rate of Cellular Aging? Cognitive Stress, Mindfulness, and Telomeres," *Annals of the New York Academy of Sciences* 1172, no. 1 (August 2009): 34–53, https://doi.org/10.1111

/j.1749-6632.2009.04414.x; and Aoife O'Donovan, A. Janet Tomiyama, Jue Lin, Eli Puterman, Nancy E. Adler, Margaret Kemeny, Owen M. Wolkowitz, Elizabeth H. Blackburn, and Elissa S. Epel, "Stress Appraisals and Cellular Aging: A Key Role for Anticipatory Threat in the Relationship between Psychological Stress and Telomere Length," *Brain, Behavior, and Immunity* 26, no. 4 (May 2012): 573–79, https://doi.org/10.1016/j.bbi.2012.01.007.

5. Jeremy P. Jamieson, Matthew K. Nock, and Wendy Berry Mendes, "Mind over Matter: Reappraising Arousal Improves Cardiovascular and Cognitive Responses to Stress," *Journal of Experimental Psychology: General* 141, no. 3 (August 2012): 417–22, https://doi.org/10.1037/a0025719.

6. Jeremy P. Jamieson, Wendy Berry Mendes, Erin Blackstock, and Toni Schmader, "Turning the Knots in Your Stomach into Bows: Reappraising Arousal Improves Performance on the GRE," *Journal of Experimental Social Psychology* 46, no. 1 (January 2010): 208–12, https://doi.org/10.1016/j.jesp.2009.08.015.

7. Alia J. Crum, Peter Salovey, and Shawn Achor, "Rethinking Stress: The Role of Mindsets in Determining the Stress Response," *Journal of Personality and Social Psychology* 104, no. 4 (April 2013): 716–33, https://doi.org/10.1037/a0031201. Items shown are adapted from Dr. Crum's Stress Mindset Measure.

8. Dena M. Bravata, Sharon A. Watts, Autumn L. Keefer, Divya K. Madhusudhan, Katie T. Taylor, Dani M. Clark, Ross S. Nelson, Kevin O. Cokley, and Heather K. Hagg. "Prevalence, Predictors, and Treatment of Impostor Syndrome: A Systematic Review," *Journal of General Internal Medicine* 35, no. 4 (April 2020): 1252–75, https://doi.org/10.1007/s11606-019-05364-1.

9. Mirjam Neureiter and Eva Traut-Mattausch, "An Inner Barrier to Career Development: Preconditions of the Impostor Phenomenon and Consequences for Career Development." *Frontiers in Psychology* 7 (February 2016): 48, https://doi.org/10.3389/fpsyg.2016.00048.

10. Patricia K. Leach, Rachel M. Nygaard, Jeffrey G. Chipman, Melissa E. Brunsvold, and Ashley P. Marek, "Impostor Phenomenon and Burnout in General Surgeons and General Surgery Residents," *Journal of Surgical Education* 76, no. 1 (2019): 99–106.

11. Özlem Ayduk and Ethan Kross, "From a Distance: Implications of Spontaneous Self-Distancing for Adaptive Self-Reflection," *Journal of Personality and Social Psychology* 98, no. 5 (May 2010): 809–29, https://doi.org/10.1037/a0019205.

12. Jenny J. W. Liu, Natalie Ein, Julia Gervasio, and Kristin Vickers, "The Efficacy of Stress Reappraisal Interventions on Stress Responsivity: A Meta-analysis and Systematic Review of Existing Evidence," *PLoS One* 14, no. 2 (February 2019): e0212854, https://doi.org/10.1371/journal.pone.0212854.

13. Jennifer Daubenmier, Elissa S. Epel, Patricia J. Moran, Jason Thompson, Ashley E. Mason, Michael Acree, Veronica Goldman, et al. "A Randomized Controlled Trial of a Mindfulness-Based Weight Loss Intervention on Cardiovascular Reactivity to Social-Evaluative Threat Among Adults with Obesity." *Mindfulness* vol. 10,12 (2019): 2583–2595. doi:10.1007/s12671-019-01232-5.

14. Kevin Love, "NBA's Kevin Love: Championing Mental Health for Everyone," Commonwealth Club, January 19, 2021, video, 1:07:31, January 27, 2021, https://www.commonwealthclub.org/events/archive/video/nbas-kevin-love -championing-mental-health-everyone.

15. Kevin Love, "Everyone Is Going through Something," *The Players' Tribune*, March 6, 2018, https://www.theplayerstribune.com/articles/kevin-love -everyone-is-going-through-something.

16. Geoffrey L. Cohen and David K. Sherman, "The Psychology of Change: Self-Affirmation and Social Psychological Intervention," *Annual Review of Psychology* 65 (January 2014): 333–71, https://doi.org/10.1146/annurev-psych -010213-115137.

17. Arghavan Salles, Claudia M. Mueller, and Geoffrey L. Cohen, "A Values Affirmation Intervention to Improve Female Residents' Surgical Performance," *Journal of Graduate Medical Education* 8, no. 3 (July 2016): 378–83, https://doi.org/10.4300/JGME-D-15-00214.1; and J. Parker Goyer, Julio Garcia, Valerie Purdie-Vaughns, Kevin R. Binning, Jonathan E. Cook, Stephanie L. Reeves, Nancy Apfel, Suzanne Taborsky-Barba, David K. Sherman, and Geoffrey L. Cohen. "Self-Affirmation Facilitates Minority Middle Schoolers' Progress along College Trajectories," *Proceedings of the National Academy of Sciences of the United States of America* 114, no. 29 (July 2017): 7594–99, https://doi.org/10.1073/pnas.1617923114.

18. J. David Creswell, Suman Lam, Annette L. Stanton, Shelley E. Taylor, Julienne E. Bower, and David K. Sherman. "Does Self-Affirmation, Cognitive Processing, or Discovery of Meaning Explain Cancer-Related Health Benefits of Expressive Writing?," *Personal and Social Psychology Bulletin* 33, no. 2 (February 2007): 238–50, https://doi.org/10.1177/0146167206294412.

19. Cohen and Sherman, "The Psychology of Change."

20. "Giving Purpose," www.givingpurpose.org/.

DAY 4: TRAIN FOR RESILIENCE

1. Elissa S. Epel, "The Geroscience Agenda: Toxic Stress, Hormetic Stress, and the Rate of Aging," *Ageing Research Reviews* 63 (November 2020): 101167, https://doi.org/10.1016/j.arr.2020.101167.

2. Caroline Kumsta, Jessica T. Chang, Jessica Schmalz, and Malene Hansen,

"Hormetic Heat Stress and HSF-1 Induce Autophagy to Improve Survival and Proteostasis in *C. elegans*," *Nature Communications* 8 (February 15, 2017): 14337, https://doi.org/10.1038/ncomms14337.

3. David G. Weissman and Wendy Berry Mendes, "Correlation of Sympathetic and Parasympathetic Nervous System Activity during Rest and Acute Stress Tasks," *International Journal of Psychophysiology* 162 (April 2021): 60–68, https://doi.org/10.1016/j.ijpsycho.2021.01.015.

4. Elissa S. Epel, Bruce S. McEwen, and Jeannette R. Ickovics, "Embodying Psychological Thriving: Physical Thriving in Response to Stress," *Journal of Social Issues* 54, no. 2 (Summer 1998): 301–22, https://doi.org/10.1111/0022-4537.671998067.

5. Manuel Mücke, Sebastian Ludyga, Flora Colledge, and Markus Gerber, "Influence of Regular Physical Activity and Fitness on Stress Reactivity as Measured with the Trier Social Stress Test Protocol: A Systematic Review," *Sports Medicine* 48, no. 11 (November 2018): 2607–22, https://doi.org/10.1007/s40279-018-0979-0.

6. Ethan L. Ostrom, Savannah R. Berry, and Tinna Traustadóttir, "Effects of Exercise Training on Redox Stress Resilience in Young and Older Adults," *Advances in Redox Research* 2 (July 2021): 10007, https://doi.org/10.1016/j.arres.2021.100007.

7. Benjamin A. Hives, E. Jean Buckler, Jordan Weiss, Samantha Schilf, Kirsten L. Johansen, Elissa S. Epel, and Eli Puterman, "The Effects of Aerobic Exercise on Psychological Functioning in Family Caregivers: Secondary Analyses of a Randomized Controlled Trial," *Annals of Behavioral Medicine* 55, no. 1 (January 2021): 65–76, https://doi.org/10.1093/abm/kaaa031.

8. Hives et al., "The Effects of Aerobic Exercise on Psychological Functioning."

9. Eli Puterman, Jordan Weiss, Jue Lin, Samantha Schilf, Aaron L. Slusher, Kirsten L. Johansen, and Elissa S. Epel. "Aerobic Exercise Lengthens Telomeres and Reduces Stress in Family Caregivers: A Randomized Controlled Trial—Curt Richter Award Paper 2018," *Psychoneuroendocrinology* 98 (December 2018): 245–52, https://doi.org/10.1016/j.psyneuen.2018.08.002.

10. Matthijs Kox, Monique Stoffels, Sanne P. Smeekens, Nens van Alfen, Marc Gomes, Thijs M. H. Eijsvogels, Maria T. E. Hopman, Johannes G. van der Hoeven, Mihai G. Netea, and Peter Pickkers, "The Influence of Concentration/Meditation on Autonomic Nervous System Activity and the Innate Immune Response: A Case Study," *Psychosomatic Medicine* 74, no. 5 (June 2012): 489–94, https://doi.org/10.1097/PSY.0b013e3182583c6d.

11. Matthijs Kox, Lucas T. van Eijk, Jelle Zwaag, Joanne van den Wildenberg, Fred C. G. J. Sweep, Johannes G. van der Hoeven, and Peter Pickkers, "Voluntary Activation of the Sympathetic Nervous System and Attenuation of

the Innate Immune Response in Humans," *Proceedings of the National Academy of Sciences of the United States of America* 111, no. 20 (May 20, 2014): 7379–84, https://doi.org/10.1073/pnas.1322174111.

12. G. A. Buijze, H. M. Y. De Jong, M. Kox, M. G. van de Sande, D. Van Schaardenburg, R. M. Van Vugt, C. D. Popa, P. Pickkers, and D. L. P. Baeten, "An Add-On Training Program Involving Breathing Exercises, Cold Exposure, and Meditation Attenuates Inflammation and Disease Activity in Axial Spondyloarthritis—a Proof of Concept Trial," *PLoS ONE* 14, no. 12 (December 2, 2019): e0225749, https://doi.org/10.1371/journal.pone.0225749.

13. Rhonda P. Patrick and Teresa L. Johnson, "Sauna Use as a Lifestyle Practice to Extend Healthspan," *Experimental Gerontology* 154 (October 15, 2021): 111509, https://doi.org/10.1016/j.exger.2021.111509.

14. Maciel Alencar Bruxel, Angela Maria Vicente Tavares, Luiz Domingues Zavarize Neto, Victor de Souza Borges, Helena Trevisan Schroeder, Patricia Martins Bock, Maria Inês Lavina Rodrigues, Adriane Belló-Klein, and Paulo Ivo Homem de Bittencourt Jr., "Chronic Whole-Body Heat Treatment Relieves Atherosclerotic Lesions, Cardiovascular and Metabolic Abnormalities, and Enhances Survival Time Restoring the Anti-inflammatory and Anti-senescent Heat Shock Response in Mice," *Biochimie* 156 (January 2019): 33–46, https://doi.org/10.1016/j.biochi.2018.09.011.

15. Kay-U. Hanusch and Clemens W. Janssen, "The Impact of Whole-Body Hyperthermia Interventions on Mood and Depression—Are We Ready for Recommendations for Clinical Application?," *International Journal of Hyperthermia* 36, no. 1 (2019): 573–81, https://doi.org/10.1080/02656736.2019.1612103.

16. Clemens W. Janssen, Christopher A. Lowry, Matthias R. Mehl, John J. B. Allen, Kimberly L. Kelly, Danielle E. Gartner, Charles L. Raison et al., "Whole-Body Hyperthermia for the Treatment of Major Depressive Disorder: A Randomized Clinical Trial," *JAMA Psychiatry* 73, no. 8 (August 1, 2016): 789–95, https://doi.org/10.1001/jamapsychiatry.2016.1031.

17. Ashley E. Mason, Sarah M. Fisher, Anoushka Chowdhary, Ekaterina Guvva, Danou Veasna, Erin Floyd, Sean B. Fender, and Charles Raison, "Feasibility and Acceptability of a Whole-Body Hyperthermia (WBH) Protocol," *International Journal of Hyperthermia* 38, no. 1 (2021): 1529–35.

DAY 5: LET NATURE DO THE WORK

1. The figures cited are from a YouGov survey of 4,382 UK adults (aged eighteen and up), May 2020, by the UK's Mental Health Foundation, which then released this helpful guide on using nature for wellness: https://www.mentalhealth.org.uk/campaigns/thriving-with-nature/guide.

2. Sarai Pouso, Ángel Borja, Lora E. Fleming, Erik Gómez-Baggethun, Mathew P. White, and María C. Uyarra, "Contact with Blue-Green Spaces during the COVID-19 Pandemic Lockdown Beneficial for Mental Health," *Science of the Total Environment* 756 (February 20, 2021): 143984, https://doi.org/10.1016/j.scitotenv.2020.143984.

3. Timothy D. Wilson, David A. Reinhard, Erin C. Westgate, Daniel T. Gilbert, Nicole Ellerbeck, Cheryl Hahn, Casey L. Brown, and Adi Shaked, "Just Think: The Challenges of the Disengaged Mind," *Science* 345, no. 6192 (July 4, 2014): 75–77, https://doi.org/10.1126/science.1250830.

4. William J. Brady, M. J. Crockett, and Jay J. Van Bavel, "The MAD Model of Moral Contagion: The Role of Motivation, Attention, and Design in the Spread of Moralized Content Online," *Perspectives on Psychological Science* 15, no. 4 (July 2020): 978–1010, https://doi.org/10.1177/1745691620917336.

5. Jeremy B. Merrill and Will Oremus, "Five Points for Anger, One for a 'Like': How Facebook's Formula Fostered Rage and Misinformation," *Washington Post*, October 26, 2021.

6. Sally C. Curtin, *State Suicide Rates among Adolescents and Young Adults Aged 10–24: United States, 2000–2018, National Vital Statistics Reports* 69, no. 11 (Hyattsville, MD: National Center for Health Statistics, 2020), 10, https://www.cdc.gov/nchs/data/nvsr/nvsr69/nvsr-69-11-508.pdf.

7. Florian Lederbogen, Peter Kirsch, Leila Haddad, Fabian Streit, Heike Tost, Philipp Schuch, Andreas Meyer-Lindenberg et al., "City Living and Urban Upbringing Affect Neural Social Stress Processing in Humans," *Nature* 474, no. 7352 (Jun 23, 2011): 498–501, https://doi.org/10.1038/nature10190.

8. Łukasz Nicewicz, Agata W. Nicewicz, Alina Kafel, and Mirosław Nakonieczny, "Set of Stress Biomarkers as a Practical Tool in the Assessment of Multistress Effect Using Honeybees from Urban and Rural Areas as a Model Organism: A Pilot Study, *Environmental Science and Pollution Research* 28, no. 8 (February 2021): 9084–96, https://doi.org/10.1007/s11356-020-11338-2.

9. Michele Antonelli, Davide Donelli, Lucrezia Carlone, Valentina Maggini, Fabio Firenzuoli, and Emanuela Bedeschi, "Effects of Forest Bathing (Shinrin-yoku) on Individual Well-Being: An Umbrella Review," *International Journal of Environmental Health Research* (April 28, 2021): 1–26, https://doi.org/10.1080/09603123.2021.1919293; and Yuki Ideno, Kunihiko Hayashi, Yukina Abe, Kayo Ueda, Hiroyasu Iso, Mitsuhiko Noda, Jung-Su Lee, and Shosuke Suzuki, "Blood Pressure-Lowering Effect of Shinrin-yoku (Forest Bathing): A Systematic Review and Meta-analysis," *BMC Complementary and Alternative Medicine* 17, no. 1 (August 16, 2017): 409, https://doi.org/10.1186/s12906-017-1912-z.

10. E. R. Jayaratne, X. Ling, and L. Morawska, "Role of Vegetation in Enhancing Radon Concentration and Ion Production in the Atmosphere," *Environmental Science & Technology* 45, no. 15 (August 1, 2011): 6350–55, https://doi.org/10.1021/es201152g.

11. Tae-Hoon Kim, Gwang-Woo Jeong, Han-Su Baek, Gwang-Won Kim, Thirunavukkarasu Sundaram, Heoung-Keun Kang, Seung-Won Lee, Hyung-Joong Kim, and Jin-Kyu Song, "Human Brain Activation in Response to Visual Stimulation with Rural and Urban Scenery Pictures: A Functional Magnetic Resonance Imaging Study," *Science of the Total Environment* 408, no. 12 (May 15, 2010): 2600–607, https://doi.org/10.1016/j.scitotenv.2010.02.025; and Simone Grassini, Antti Revonsuo, Serena Castellotti, Irene Petrizzo, Viola Benedetti, and Mika Koivisto, "Processing of Natural Scenery Is Associated with Lower Attentional and Cognitive Load Compared with Urban Ones," *Journal of Environmental Psychology* 62 (April 2019): 1–11, https://doi.org/10.1016/j.jenvp.2019.01.007.

12. Pooja Sahni and Jyoti Kumar, "Effect of Nature Experience on Frontoparietal Correlates of Neurocognitive Processes Involved in Directed Attention: An ERP Study," *Annals of Neurosciences* 27, no. 3–4 (July 2020): 136–47, https://doi.org/10.1177/0972753121990143.

13. Justin S. Feinstein, Sahib S. Khalsa, Hung Yeh, Obada Al Zoubi, Armen C. Arevian, Colleen Wohlrab, Martin P. Paulus et al., "The Elicitation of Relaxation and Interoceptive Awareness Using Floatation Therapy in Individuals with High Anxiety Sensitivity," *Biological Psychiatry: Cognitive Neuroscience and Neuroimaging* 3, no. 6 (June 2018): 555–62, https://doi.org/10.1016/j.bpsc.2018.02.005; and Justin S. Feinstein, Sahib S. Khalsa, Hung-Wen Yeh, Colleen Wohlrab, W. Kyle Simmons, Murray B. Stein, and Martin P. Paulus, "Examining the Short-Term Anxiolytic and Antidepressant Effect of Floatation-REST," *PLoS One* 13, no. 2 (February 2, 2018): e0190292, https://doi.org/10.1371/journal.pone.0190292.

14. Virginia Sturm, Samir Datta, Ashlin Roy, Isabel Sible, Eena Kosik, Christina Veziris, Tiffany E. Chow et al., "Big Smile, Small Self: Awe Walks Promote Prosocial Positive Emotions in Older Adults," *Emotion* (September 21, 2020) [Epub ahead of print]. doi: 10.1037/emo0000876: http://dx.doi.org/10.1037/emo0000876.

15. "Stress & Resilience with Elissa Epel and Dacher Keltner," *City Arts & Lectures*, KQED, May 11, 2021, 1:06:09, www.cityarts.net/event/stress-resilience/.

16. Michelle C. Kondo, Jaime M. Fluehr, Thomas McKeon, and Charles C. Branas, "Urban Green Space and Its Impact on Human Health," *International Journal of Environmental Research and Public Health* 15, no. 3 (March 2018): 445, https://doi.org/10.3390/ijerph15030445.

17. Gert-Jan Vanaken and Marina Danckaerts, "Impact of Green Space Exposure on Children's and Adolescents' Mental Health: A Systematic Review," *International Journal of Environmental Research and Public Health* 5, no. 12 (December 2018): 2668, https://doi.org/10.3390/ijerph15122668.

18. Jean Woo et al. "Green Space, Psychological Restoration, and Telomere Length." *The Lancet* 373, no. 9660 (January 2009): 299–300, https://doi.org/10.1016/S0140-6736(09)60094-5.

19. Noëlie Molbert, Frédéric Angelier, Fabrice Alliot, Cécile Ribout, and Aurélie Goutte, "Fish from Urban Rivers and with High Pollutant Levels Have Shorter Telomeres," *Biology Letters* 17, no. 1 (January 2021): 20200819, https://doi.org/10.1098/rsbl.2020.0819.

20. Juan Diego Ibáñez-Álamo, Javier Pineda-Pampliega, Robert L. Thomson, José I. Aguirre, Alazne Díez-Fernández, Bruno Faivre, Jordi Figuerola, and Simon Verhulst, "Urban Blackbirds Have Shorter Telomeres," *Biology Letters* 14, no. 3 (March 2018): 20180083, https://doi.org/10.1098/rsbl.2018.0083.

21. Mark Coleman, *Awake in the Wild: Mindfulness in Nature as a Path of Self-Discovery* (Maui, HI: Inner Ocean Publishing, 2006)

22. Thich Nhat Hanh, *Peace Is Every Step* (New York: Bantam Books, 1992).

23. Brian Cooke and Edzard Ernst, "Aromatherapy: A Systematic Review," *British Journal of General Practice* 50, no. 455 (June 2000): 493–96, https://bjgp.org/content/50/455/493.long; and Hyun-Ju Kang, Eun Sook Nam, Yongmi Lee, and Myoungsuk Kim, "How Strong Is the Evidence for the Anxiolytic Efficacy of Lavender?: Systematic Review and Meta-analysis of Randomized Controlled Trials," *Asian Nursing Research* 13, no. 5 (December 2019): 295–305, https://doi.org/10.1016/j.anr.2019.11.003.

24. Timothy K. H. Fung, Benson W. M. Lau, Shirley P. C. Ngai, and Hector W. H. Tsang, "Therapeutic Effect and Mechanisms of Essential Oils in Mood Disorders: Interaction between the Nervous and Respiratory Systems," *International Journal of Molecular Sciences* 22, no. 9 (May 1, 2021): 4844, https://doi.org/10.3390/ijms22094844.

25. John Muir, *Our National Parks* (San Francisco: Sierra Club Books, 1991).

26. Shigehiro Oishi, Thomas Talhelm, and Minha Lee, "Personality and Geography: Introverts Prefer Mountains," *Journal of Research in Personality* 58 (October 2015): 55–68, https://doi.org/10.1016/j.jrp.2015.07.001.

DAY 6: DON'T JUST RELAX . . . RESTORE

1. James Nestor, *Breath: The New Science of a Lost Art* (New York: Riverhead Books, 2020).

2. Lisa Feldman Barrett, "The Theory of Constructed Emotion: An Active Inference Account of Interoception and Categorization," *Social Cognitive and Affective Neuroscience* 12, no. 1 (January 2017): 1–23, https://doi.org/10.1093/scan/nsw154.

3. E. S. Epel, E. Puterman, J. Lin, E. H. Blackburn, P. Y. Lum, N. D. Beckmann, E. E. Schadt et al., "Meditation and Vacation Effects Have an Impact on Disease-Associated Molecular Phenotypes," *Translational Psychiatry* 6, no. 8 (August 2016): e880, https://doi.org/10.1038/tp.2016.164.

4. Shannon Harvey, *My Year of Living Mindfully* (Sydney: Hachette Australia, 2020).

5. Stefanie E. Mayer, Agus Surachman, Aric A. Prather, Eli Puterman, Kevin L. Delucchi, Michael R. Irwin, Andrea Danese, David M. Almeida, and Elissa S. Epel, "The Long Shadow of Childhood Trauma for Depression in Midlife: Examining Daily Psychological Stress Processes as a Persistent Risk Pathway," *Psychological Medicine* (March 26, 2021): 1–10, https://doi.org/10.1017/S0033291721000921.

6. Xiaoli Chen, Rui Wang, Phyllis Zee, Pamela L. Lutsey, Sogol Javaheri, Carmela Alcántara, Chandra L. Jackson, Michelle A. Williams, and Susan Redline, "Racial/Ethnic Differences in Sleep Disturbances: The Multi-ethnic Study of Atherosclerosis (MESA)," *Sleep* 38, no. 6 (June 1, 2015): 877–88, https://doi.org/10.5665/sleep.4732.

7. Tricia Hersey, *Rest Is Resistance: A Manifesto* (New York: Little, Brown Spark, 2022).

8. Nestor, *Breath*.

9. Patrick McKeown, *The Breathing Cure: Develop New Habits for a Healthier, Happier, and Longer Life* (New York: Humanix Books, 2021).

10. Andrea Zaccaro, Andrea Piarulli, Marco Laurino, Erika Garbella, Danilo Menicucci, Bruno Neri, and Angelo Gemignani, "How Breath-Control Can Change Your Life: A Systematic Review on Psycho-physiological Correlates of Slow Breathing," *Frontiers in Human Neuroscience* 12 (September 7, 2018): 353, https://doi.org/10.3389/fnhum.2018.00353.

11. Mikołaj Tytus Szulczewski, "An Anti-hyperventilation Instruction Decreases the Drop in End-Tidal CO_2 and Symptoms of Hyperventilation during Breathing at 0.1 Hz," *Applied Psychophysiology and Biofeedback* 44, no. 3 (September 2019): 247–56, https://doi.org/10.1007/s10484-019-09438-y; Paul Lehrer, E. Vaschillo, and Bronya Vaschillo, "Resonant Frequency Biofeedback Training to Increase Cardiac Variability: Rationale and Manual for Training," *Applied Psychophysiology and Biofeedback* 25, no. 3 (2000): 177–191.

12. Juliana M. B. Khoury, Margo C. Watt, and Kim MacLean, "Anxiety Sensitivity Mediates Relations between Mental Distress Symptoms and Medical

Care Utilization during COVID-19 Pandemic," *International Journal of Cognitive Therapy* 14, no. 3 (September 2021): 515–36, https://doi.org/10.1007/s41811-021-00113-x.

13. Alicia E. Meuret, Frank H. Wilhelm, Thomas Ritz, and Walton T. Roth, "Feedback of End-Tidal pCO_2 as a Therapeutic Approach for Panic Disorder," *Journal of Psychiatric Research* 42, no. 7 (June 2008): 560–68, https://doi.org/10.1016/j.jpsychires.2007.06.005.

DAY 7: START FULL, END FULL

1. Jennifer R. Piazza, Susan T. Charles, Martin J. Sliwinski, Jacqueline Mogle, and David M. Almeida, "Affective Reactivity to Daily Stressors and Long-Term Risk of Reporting a Chronic Physical Health Condition," *Annals of Behavioral Medicine* 45, no. 1 (February 2013): 110–20, https://doi.org/10.1007/s12160-012-9423-0; and Daniel K. Mroczek, Robert S. Stawski, Nicholas A. Turiano, Wai Chan, David M. Almeida, Shevaun D. Neupert, and Avron Spiro III, "Emotional Reactivity and Mortality: Longitudinal Findings from the VA Normative Aging Study," *Journals of Gerontology: Series B* 70, no. 3 (May 2015): 398–406. https://doi.org/10.1093/geronb/gbt107.

2. K. Aschbacher, E. Epel, O. M. Wolkowitz, A. A. Prather, E. Puterman, and F. S. Dhabhar, "Maintenance of a Positive Outlook during Acute Stress Protects against Pro-inflammatory Reactivity and Future Depressive Symptoms," *Brain, Behavior, and Immunity* 26, no. 2 (February 2012): 346–52, https://doi.org/10.1016/j.bbi.2011.10.010.

3. Judith T. Moskowitz, Elizabeth L. Addington, and Elaine O. Cheung, "Positive Psychology and Health: Well-Being Interventions in the Context of Illness," *General Hospital Psychiatry* 61 (November–December 2019): 136–38, https://doi.org/10.1016/j.genhosppsych.2019.11.001.

4. Eric L. Garland, Barbara Fredrickson, Ann M. Kring, David P. Johnson, Piper S. Meyer, and David L. Penn, "Upward Spirals of Positive Emotions Counter Downward Spirals of Negativity: Insights from the Broaden-and-Build Theory and Affective Neuroscience on the Treatment of Emotion Dysfunctions and Deficits in Psychopathology," *Clinical Psychology Review* 30, no 7 (November 2010): 849–64, https://doi.org/10.1016/j.cpr.2010.03.002.

5. Judith T. Moskowitz, Elaine O. Cheung, Karin E. Snowberg, Alice Verstaen, Jennifer Merrilees, John M. Salsman, and Glenna A. Dowling, "Randomized Controlled Trial of a Facilitated Online Positive Emotion Regulation Intervention for Dementia Caregivers," *Health Psychology* 38, no. 5 (May 2019): 391–402, https://doi.org/10.1037/hea0000680.

6. Barbara Fredrickson, "The Broaden-and-Build Theory of Positive Emo-

tions," *Philosophical Transactions of the Royal Society B* 359, no. 1449 (September 29, 2004): 1367–78, https://doi.org/10.1098/rstb.2004.1512.

7. Dusti R. Jones and Jennifer E. Graham-Engeland, "Positive Affect and Peripheral Inflammatory Markers among Adults: A Narrative Review," *Psychoneuroendocrinology* 123 (January 2021): 104892, https://doi.org/10.1016/j.psyneuen.2020.104892.

8. Sheldon Cohen, William J. Doyle, Ronald B. Turner, Cuneyt M. Alper, and David P. Skoner, "Emotional Style and Susceptibility to the Common Cold," *Psychosomatic Medicine* 65, no. 4 (July–August 2003): 652–57, https://doi.org/10.1097/01.psy.0000077508.57784.da.

9. Yujing Zhang and Buxin Han, "Positive Affect and Mortality Risk in Older Adults: A Meta-analysis," *Psychology Journal* 5, no. 2 (June 2016): 125–38, https://doi.org/10.1002/pchj.129.

10. Tsoknyi Rinpoche, *Open Heart, Open Mind: Awakening the Power of Essence Love* (New York: Harmony Books, 2012). This book describes in more detail the Handshake with Emotion and other practices that promote inner joy.

11. Anthony D. Ong, Lizbeth Benson, Alex J. Zautra, and Nilam Ram, "Emodiversity and Biomarkers of Inflammation," *Emotion* 18, no. 1 (February 2018): 3–14, https://doi.org/10.1037/emo0000343; and E. J. Urban-Wojcik, J. A. Mumford, D. M. Almeida, M. E. Lachman, C. D. Ryff, R. J. Davidson, and S. M. Schaefer, "Emodiversity, Health, and Well-Being in the Midlife in the United States (MIDUS) Daily Diary Study," *Emotion* (April 9, 2020): https://doi.org/10.1037/emo0000753.

12. Inês M. Tavares, Hera E. Schlagintweit, Pedro J. Nobre, and Natalie O. Rosen, "Sexual Well-Being and Perceived Stress in Couples Transitioning to Parenthood: A Dyadic Analysis," *International Journal of Clinical and Health Psychology* 19, no. 3 (September 2019): 198–208, https://doi.org/10.1016/j.ijchp.2019.07.004.

13. Andrea Burri and Ana Carvalheira, "Masturbatory Behavior in a Population Sample of German Women," *Journal of Sexual Medicine* 16, no. 7 (July 2019): 963–74, https://doi.org/10.1016/j.jsxm.2019.04.015.

14. Esther Perel, "Why Eroticism Should Be Part of Your Self-Care Plan," *Esther Perel* (blog), accessed May 17, 2022, https://www.estherperel.com/blog/eroticism-self-care-plan.

15. Robert H. Lustig, *The Hacking of the American Mind: The Science Behind the Corporate Takeover of Our Bodies and Brains* (New York: Avery, 2017).

16. June Gruber, Aleksandr Kogan, Jordi Quoidbach, and Iris B. Mauss, "Happiness Is Best Kept Stable: Positive Emotion Variability Is Associated with Poorer Psychological Health, *Emotion* 13, no. 1 (February 2013): 1–6, https://doi.org/10.1037/a0030262.

17. Peter Koval, Barbara Ogrinz, Peter Kuppens, Omer Van den Bergh, Francis Tuerlinckx, and Stefan Sütterlin, "Affective Instability in Daily Life Is Predicted by Resting Heart Rate Variability," *PLoS One* 8, no. 11 (November 29, 2013): e81536, https://doi.org/10.1371/journal.pone.0081536.

18. Anthony D. Ong and Andrew Steptoe, "Association of Positive Affect Instability with All-Cause Mortality in Older Adults in England," *JAMA Network Open* 3, no. 7 (July 1, 2020): e207725, https://doi.org/10.1001/jamanetwork open.2020.7725.

19. Lustig, *The Hacking of the American Mind*.

20. Kennon M. Sheldon and Sonja Lyubomirsky, "Revisiting the Sustainable Happiness Model and Pie Chart: Can Happiness Be Successfully Pursued?," *Journal of Positive Psychology* 16, no. 2 (2021): 145–54, https://doi.org/10 .1080/17439760.2019.1689421.

21. S. Katherine Nelson, Kristin Layous, Steven W. Cole, and Sonja Lyubomirsky, "Do unto Others or Treat Yourself? The Effects of Prosocial and Self-Focused Behavior on Psychological Flourishing," *Emotion* 16, no. 6 (September 2016): 850–61, https://doi.org/10.1037/emo0000178.

22. S. Katherine Nelson-Coffey, Megan M. Fritz, Sonja Lyubomirsky, and Steve W. Cole, "Kindness in the Blood: A Randomized Controlled Trial of the Gene Regulatory Impact of Prosocial Behavior," *Psychoneuroendocrinology* 81 (July 2017): 8–13, https://doi.org/10.1016/j.psyneuen.2017.03.025.

23. Kuan-Hua Chen, Casey L. Brown, Jenna L. Wells, Emily S. Rothwell, Marcela C. Otero, Robert W. Levenson, and Barbara L Fredrickson, "Physiological Linkage during Shared Positive and Shared Negative Emotion," *Journal of Personality and Social Psychology* 121, no. 5 (November 2021): 10.1037 /pspi0000337, https://doi.org/10.1037/pspi0000337; Jenna Wells, Claudia Haase, Emily Rothwell, Kendyl Naugle, Marcela Otero, Casey Brown, Jocelyn Lai et al., "Positivity Resonance in Long-Term Married Couples: Multimodal Characteristics and Consequences for Health and Longevity," *Journal of Personality and Social Psychology* (January 31, 2022), https://doi.org/10 .1037/pspi0000385.

24. Jaime Vila, "Social Support and Longevity: Meta-Analysis-Based Evidence and Psychobiological Mechanisms," *Frontiers in Psychology* 12 (September 13, 2021), https://doi.org/10.3389/fpsyg.2021.717164.; and Ted Robles, Richard Slatcher, Joseph Trombello, and Mehgan McGinn, "Marital Quality and Health: A Meta-analytic Review," *Psychological Bulletin* 140, no 1 (January 2014): 140–87. https://10.1037/a0031859.

25. Nicholas A. Coles, Jeff T. Larsen, and Heather C. Lench, "A Meta-analysis of the Facial Feedback Literature: Effects of Facial Feedback on Emotional Experience Are Small and Variable," *Psychological Bulletin* 145, no. 6 (June

2019): 610–55, https://doi.org/10.1037/bul0000194; Nicholas A. Coles, David Scott March, Fernando Marmolejo-Ramos, Jeff T. Larsen, Nwadiogo C. Chisom Arinze, Izuchukwu L. G. Ndukaihe, Megan L. Willis et al., "A Multi-lab Test of the Facial Feedback Hypothesis by the Many Smiles Collaboration," *PsyArXiv Preprints* (February 4, 2019): 1–54, https://doi.org/10.31234/osf.io /cvpuw.

26. Pennie Eddy, Eleanor H. Wertheim, Matthew W. Hale, and Bradley J. Wright, "A Systematic Review and Meta-analysis of the Effort-Reward Imbalance Model of Workplace Stress and Hypothalamic-Pituitary-Adrenal Axis Measures of Stress," *Psychosomatic Medicine* 80, no. 1 (January 2018): 103–13, https://doi.org/10.1097/PSY.0000000000000505.

27. Martin Picard, Aric A. Prather, Eli Puterman, Kirstin Aschbacher, Yan Burelle, and Elissa S. Epel, "A Mitochondrial Health Index Sensitive to Mood and Caregiving Stress," *Biological Psychiatry* 84, no. 1 (July 1, 2018): 9–17, https://doi.org/10.1016/j.biopsych.2018.01.012.

28. Christina Armenta, Megan Fritz, Lisa Walsh, and Sonja Lyubomirsky, "Satisfied Yet Striving: Gratitude Fosters Life Satisfaction and Improvement Motivation in Youth," *Emotion* (September 10, 2020): https://doi.org /10.1037/emo0000896.

CONCLUSION

1. Daniel J. Siegel, IntraConnected: *MWe (Me + We) as the Integration of Self, Identity, and Belonging (IPNB)* (New York: W. W. Norton & Company, 2022).

2. Shantideva, *The Way of the Bodhisattva* (Boston: Shambhala, 2006), chapter 8, verse 129.

3. "Embracing Hope, Courage, and Compassion in Times of Crisis," His Holiness the 14th Dalai Lama of Tibet, December 8, 2021, https://www.dalailama .com/news/2021/embracing-hope-courage-and-compassion-in-times-of -crisis

4. Pádraig Ó Tuama, Daily Prayer with the Corrymeela Community (Norwich, UK: Canterbury Press, 2017).

5. Karen O'Brien, *You Matter More Than You Think: Quantum Social Change for a Thriving World* (Oslo, Norway: cChange Press, 2021).

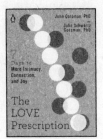

THE LOVE PRESCRIPTION

Seven Days to More Intimacy, Connection, and Joy

For the past forty years, Drs. John Gottman and Julie Schwartz Gottman have been studying love. They've gathered data on over three thousand couples, looking at everything from their body language to the way they converse to their stress hormone levels. Their goal: identify the building blocks of love.

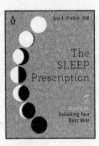

THE SLEEP PRESCRIPTION

Seven Days to Unlocking Your Best Rest

Sleep is as essential as food, water, and oxygen. So how can something that should be so instinctual and automatic be so hard? Dr. Aric Prather runs one of the world's most successful sleep clinics and has cracked the code to help even the most restless of sleepers get a good night's rest.

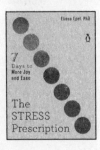

THE STRESS PRESCRIPTION

Seven Days to More Joy and Ease

While we can't eliminate stress altogether, what we *can* change is our response to it. Dr. Elissa Epel has dedicated her career to studying stress. And what she's learned over years of research is that the secret to tackling stress is not simply to avoid it—it's to experience stress *differently*.

 PENGUIN BOOKS

Ready to find your next great read? Let us help. Visit prh.com/nextread